FINDING RESILIENCE THROUGH

G.R.A.C.E.

FROM CANCER DIAGNOSIS TO EMPOWERMENT

Jody Ford, PhD

Finding Resilience Through
G.R.A.C.E.
From Cancer Diagnosis to Empowerment

© 2026 Jody Ford, PhD

Published by Jody Ford
Elkhorn, Nebraska

Library of Congress Control Number: 2026906547
ISBN: 979-8-9949102-0-7

Subjects:
HEA039030 HEALTH & FITNESS / Diseases & Conditions / Cancer
BIO017000 BIOGRAPHY & AUTOBIOGRAPHY / Medical
MED011000 MEDICAL / Caregiving

Cover Design by Ashley Spitsnogle
Interior and Back Cover Design by Brian Schroeder © 2026.

"This book is a lifeline. Through raw honesty and thoughtful guidance, the author offers more than her story—she offers structure and strength for anyone navigating the emotional terrain of cancer. Having lost loved ones to this disease and stood beside survivors in their fight, I know how rare it is to find something both deeply human and genuinely practical. This is a must-read for every patient, survivor, and caregiver searching for steadiness in uncertain ground."

– Shawn D. Kuenzi, MS

Senior Human Resources Leader | Strategic Workforce Planning | Organizational Development

"Jody Ford poignantly describes her deeply personal cancer journey using knowledge, compassion, and humor. *Finding Resilience through G.R.A.C.E.* is a guide not only for those who are going through their own health journey, but also for caregivers who want to try to understand and help in meaningful ways. A book I wish I had earlier, and one to be read more than once."

– Rebecca Winterfeld, MA

Educational Counseling and Psychology

"*Finding Resilience through G.R.A.C.E.* is a masterclass in translating professional expertise into personal survival techniques. As a leader and former colleague, I've always admired Jody's hunger for growth and her tenacity in the face of challenges. Here, she applies her same relentlessness and creativity to the chaos of a dual cancer diagnosis. While many books offer either advice or inspiration, this guide provides both. By weaving her vulnerable, in-the-trenches journey with the actionable G.R.A.C.E. framework and reflective self-coaching exercises, Jody helps readers navigate the unpredictable and rough waters of cancer. This is an essential resource for patients and caregivers seeking a structured, honest, and highly practical roadmap to reclaiming their agency when life feels unrecognizable."

– Rebecca Crotts, MS

Organizational Dynamics | Organizational Consulting | Executive Coaching

"Jody Ford is one of the most resilient women I know, and her strong sense of purpose and giving nature are evident throughout this book. Having many family members and friends impacted by cancer, I can't help but wish we'd had this book to guide us through its complexities and chaos. The practical and relatable strategies laid out in this book will no doubt help many others navigate cancers challenges."

– Jodi Maciejewski,

Enterprise Project and Change Management

"Turning pain into a path forward is something very precious and challenging. This book will help you consider options and take care of yourself so you can move forward with GRACE."

– Nina Swanson, MS

Labor and Industrial Relations | Training | Organization Development

Dedicated to my friends and family

Because of you, I found the strength to keep going …

and the courage to write this book.

ACKNOWLEDGEMENTS

TO MY HUSBAND, JEFF, WHO lived the promise of "in sickness and in health." When I could not make decisions, you made them with courage. When the road became unbearably hard, you never left my side. Your devotion as my caregiver, advocate, and partner carried me through more obstacles than either one of us imagined we would experience.

To my brother, Rusty, and his wife, Bridget, for the countless miles you traveled to be there for Jeff and me during this journey. You helped carry the burden of difficult decisions and advocated for me when I could not. Each time you walked into my hospital room, a sense of calm and reassurance followed. Your presence reminded me of the importance of family.

To Rebecca C., Rebecca W., Nina, Shawn, and Jodi who committed time to read this work and share your thoughtful insights—a simple thank you doesn't seem enough. Your encouragement, honesty, and perspective helped shape this book in meaningful ways, and I am deeply grateful for your contributions and support.

To my amazing community, of whom there are too many to mention here, but you know who you are. You stepped forward, without prompting, when I needed you most. You cared for me when I was at my weakest, sat quietly beside me as I drifted in and out of consciousness, and traveled from near and far simply to be present. In moments when words were unnecessary, your compassion, patience, and steady presence brought comfort and strength. You made my journey tolerable and my recovery possible.

Lastly, I am forever in debt to the brilliant medical teams who were my guides for this journey. Without them, I wouldn't be here. They are unsung heroes and models of expertise and compassion.

$$G.$$ oogle with Purpose, Not Panic

$$R.$$ esist the Advice Avalanche

$$A.$$ cknowledge the Emotional Roller Coaster

$$C.$$ ling to Your Community

$$E.$$ mbrace Your New Normal

TABLE OF CONTENTS

RESOURCES

INTRODUCTION

"We shouldn't pray for an easy life, but the strength to endure a difficult one."
– Father Stu (Movie with Mark Wahlberg)

MY LIFE STORY IS ONE OF EXCITEMENT and adventure. I've been blessed at almost every turn and graced with good fortune with years of well-being, a great network of friends, and family members who have always been there for me. Since I was young, I've had a strong sense of purpose and spent most of my life striving to achieve all I could. My world, as I knew it, changed on August 4, 2021. That's the day I became a member of the breast cancer club, a club no one ever wants to join. My wonderful world took a detour, and it would take over four years to navigate what was a very scary journey.

Why this guide? Because my purpose on this earth isn't over yet. And my experiences were all opportunities to learn, regardless of how painful or challenging they were. Throughout my professional career, I've focused on helping others learn and grow, and this cancer journey allowed me to learn many new lessons and apply some of the knowledge gleaned from my professional work and studies.

So many women whom I've had discussions with say, "I didn't hear a thing after the doctor said, 'you have breast cancer.'" This happened to me. I was driving down the I-5 freeway in Los Angeles when my doctor called. All I heard after "cancer" was "triple-negative breast cancer" and "rare and aggressive." I'm so lucky I didn't cause a wreck!

The first thing I did was go home and Google triple-negative breast cancer (TNBC). I don't know how I got along for so many years without Dr. Google! Sure enough, it is a rare and aggressive type of breast cancer that spreads and grows quickly, impacting only 10-15 percent of all breast cancer cases. It's unique because effective treatments for other types of breast cancer are not as effective against TNBC. I kept reading, and the sobs I'd been holding in were quickly preparing to erupt. Statistically the odds are stacked against triple-negative patients, and I specifically remember the website saying there was a 20-30 percent five-year survival rate for advanced stages of TNBC. I immediately thought, *I'm going to die soon!* Had I kept reading, I would have seen that the five-year survival rate is around 77 percent overall, and I could have saved my tears for a later time. Heck, I didn't even know the stage of my cancer.

Following seven rounds of chemotherapy, each taking seven and a half hours, five weeks of daily radiation, and a partial mastectomy, tests showed we had achieved a complete recovery. My surgeon told me this is not very common. Woohoo! I had beaten the odds!

Even though I celebrated this news with much elation, I still had a nagging feeling in the back of my mind that I was not truly through with this journey. You see, the online articles Google led me to also said there was a 40 percent risk of recurrence for early-stage TNBC. I took all this to heart, and it was the scariest time of my life.

I never felt like I fully recovered because fatigue and shortness of breath continued to be my adversaries. These were two of the side effects from going through the previous treatments, so no one seemed too concerned. But my body was telling me it was not okay. Ten months after my final immunotherapy treatment, I was back at the oncologist, and that's when the second shock wave hit.

Following blood labs and a bone marrow biopsy, I was diagnosed with blood cancer. A bone marrow biopsy is taken from the back through the hip bone. A drill is used to create a hole in the bone—yes, a drill like one you'd find in most toolboxes—and fluid and tissue are sucked out for the biopsy. Was the area numbed? Yes. But numbing doesn't work on bone. Of all the needles, medications, you name it … this was the MOST painful process I encountered. By the fourth biopsy, I was at least prepared when I heard the whirring of the drill.

My biopsy results were diagnosed as myelodysplastic syndrome (MDS), a rare group of bone marrow failure disorders where the body no longer makes enough healthy, normal blood cells in the bone marrow. In discussions with various medical team members, this incurable blood cancer was more than likely the result of all the chemotherapy and radiation treatments for TNBC. (I'm hitting the lottery on rare cancers by now.) No wonder I was tired all the time and couldn't catch my breath! My red blood cells couldn't produce and transport enough oxygen from my lungs to tissues throughout my body to produce energy.

I immediately began chemotherapy treatments, and the wheels were put in motion to have an allogeneic (someone else's cells) stem cell transplant. Fortunately for me, I live just a few miles from one of the leading stem cell transplant hospitals in the nation and I felt confident in the medical team that took on my case.

The bigger hurdle was finding an allogeneic donor match for my transplant. Unfortunately, my brother was not a match. Friends came out of the woodwork and offered to be tested to help me out. I was humbled by the outpouring of people who stepped forward to donate to my cause. However, desired transplant donors are between the ages of eighteen and forty, so I had the task of letting many of them know they were considered too old to be a donor. I might have had a few chuckles delivering this message to some, but I'll never admit it. I made a commitment to myself early on to find humor in my journey. It was either laugh or cry, and I chose to laugh as much as I could.

My donor was one of four who showed as a possible match in the international database, World Marrow Donor Association (WMDA). My donor was a thirty-four-year-old female living outside of the United States, and because of HIPAA and other confidentiality agreements, I received no further information about her.

Words can't express the gratitude I have for her willingness to help save a life; my life. And just in case you're wondering, there is a three-year waiting period for us to decide whether we want our information shared with the other. I'm still less than three years into this, so I have time to make my decision.

Prior to my stem cell transplant I spent two weeks in quarantine at the hospital where I went through a preparative regimen consisting of chemotherapy and full-body radiation. The purpose of this was to destroy as many of the diseased cells in my body as possible, and to weaken my immune system to keep my body from rejecting the donated cells after transplant.

On December 21, 2023, referred to as Day Zero in the transplant world, my stem cells arrived by airplane, and we were given the go-ahead to start the transplant. This day is called a birthday because it's like the beginning of a new life. My son and a dear friend (the same one who was there for my first chemo treatment and throughout my ordeal) were both present for moral support. Unfortunately, my husband was exposed to COVID-19 and needed to stay as far away from me as possible. To dispel any rumors you may have heard, a stem-cell transplant is really a non-event because it's just like getting a blood transfusion. No pain. No special equipment. Very anti-climactic physically … at least during the transfusion.

The medical team did a great job of preparing me for the post-transplant activities and the possible side effects I could encounter, the most crucial being graft versus host disease (GVHD). This side effect is caused when the transplanted immune cells (graft) attack the recipient's body (host). I was not prepared for GVHD to be the culprit of my biggest challenge. All along, I thought it would be the cancer that would kill me.

It's normal to have GVHD, and somewhat of a good sign because it indicates that the new cells are attacking the old cells. Mine came in the form of a skin rash. In retrospect, we had plenty of education about it possibly taking up to one year to recover and feel better, but we never discussed what a worst-case scenario of GVHD could do to my body. One of the first of many lessons learned about having a serious disease.

Before I go any further, I'd like to share a fact that most people aren't aware of and it's kind of fun to watch people's expressions when I tell them about this medical phenomenon. The allogeneic stem cell transplant totally wiped out my existing DNA and blood type, and today, my DNA and blood type are those of my donor. It's like taking a computer hard drive and wiping it clean to install an all-new operating system.

After a few weeks in the hospital, I was able to return home to recover. After about one week at home, I noticed a merlot-colored rash on my arms that quickly spread to my legs. It itched. Oh my gosh it itched! And it became painful. The doctor prescribed topical creams, and nothing worked. The itching became unbearable, and eventually it was time to go to the hospital to find relief. The rash quickly spread and was soon on my torso. Blisters and rash soon covered me from head to toe! It never crossed our minds that it would be four months before I would return home.

I don't recall much after being taken to the hospital and admitted into the intensive care unit for acute GVHD. The pain medications numbed my brain. I'm told, and the pictures validate, that much of my skin blistered and peeled off, much like I had suffered severe burns. Some of my skin became thick and sharp-edged, and I managed to scratch and damage my eyelids and the corneas of my eyes.

My wounds needed constant monitoring and cleaning to avoid infection. I do recall screaming and crying because it hurt so much when the nurses worked on replacing the gauze wrapping my body. My doctors presented options for treatment to my husband and family. Fly me to the closest burn unit hospital or put me into a medically induced coma to manage the pain. I'm told that the doctor asked me what I wanted to do, and I responded, "Do whatever it takes." Within minutes, they had me in a medically induced coma, and I remained sedated for nine days.

If you've ever wondered if there is brain activity in the mind of a coma patient, my answer is yes. Kind of. I experienced some of the wildest hallucinations one could imagine. It was difficult to distinguish what was reality and what was a hallucination. My thinking was a blur. The underlying theme to every storyline in my mind was me trying to escape the pain that was inflicted on me. I have recollections of screaming, crying, and yelling when they changed my dressings. All the while, I was trying to figure out how to escape this hell. I constantly felt exhausted as I was trying to get away from the people who were drugging me and "tying me down."

When I became coherent, the reality set in that I was not tied down; my muscles no longer functioned. Having lain in a hospital bed for a little over six weeks, muscle atrophy had set in. I recognized the faces of my nurses—the bad people from my hallucinations who kept drugging me and putting me to sleep. Later, my husband told me that when I started to stir and come out of the coma, they would sedate me again, so part of my hallucinations were real.

For four weeks, give or take, everything was a blur. My inability to move at all was a harsh reality and probably the most difficult psychological barrier to overcome. Having my body restricted to a prone position had not been part of my mental preparation for this transplant. In fact, it was traumatizing when I started to realize what was going on. Unfortunately, the morphine and other drugs prevented me from thinking clearly enough to understand that someday, I would once again be able to sit and walk. At the time, I thought I was going to be a paraplegic for the rest of my life. I had lost control of every muscle in my body except for my ability to speak and open my eyes. The anger I felt grew every day, and a few times, I believed I wanted life to be over. The question I kept asking myself was *do I have it in me to overcome this?*

Once I was well enough to leave the hospital, I was transferred to a rehabilitation facility to undergo physical therapy. I was confined to a wheelchair and, by then, I had begun to build up strength in my arms. Trying to feed myself was still a challenge and was deemed entertaining to my spouse, especially when I tried to eat a banana and kept missing my mouth. After a long, grueling six weeks of intense physical therapy learning how to do what I had taken for granted my whole life, I went home on April 19, 2024.

Still reliant on a walker and wheelchair, I continued working on my ability to walk and climb stairs and rebuild the muscles that so quickly deteriorated. I have a true appreciation now for having the ability to sit, stand, walk, go to the bathroom by myself, and the list goes on. I struggled emotionally and psychologically going from a very independent woman to one of complete dependence.

Today, I lead a fairly normal life. My new normal, though, is a far cry from what used to be normal for me. Brain fog still plagues me, and it took about fourteen months before I started feeling better. Those fourteen months were filled with more than 350 doctor visits, with some weeks having four days of appointments. I experienced many ups and downs and slept a lot during this time.

So here I am. It's been a long, hard journey. Along the way, I've learned so much about myself, about others, and life in general. Hence the title. I learned to be resilient during the toughest of times, and what I believe got me through it all was GRACE. Forget about the medical stuff. I learned how to distill everything into what is and isn't important in life. Thus, the motivation to write this book. My goal is to share some stories, provide ideas on how to turn chaos into calm, and suggest ways for you to take control of your journey instead of your journey controlling you.

This is my story. What I've endured may or may not be riveting to read about; however, I do know that some of what I experienced put me in a unique group. I hope this book inspires you to never give up on yourself. To be aware of the potential hazards that can set you back psychologically. And lastly, to know that no matter how hard life becomes, you should never give up on yourself.

Read.

Reflect.

Laugh.

Cry.

Hope.

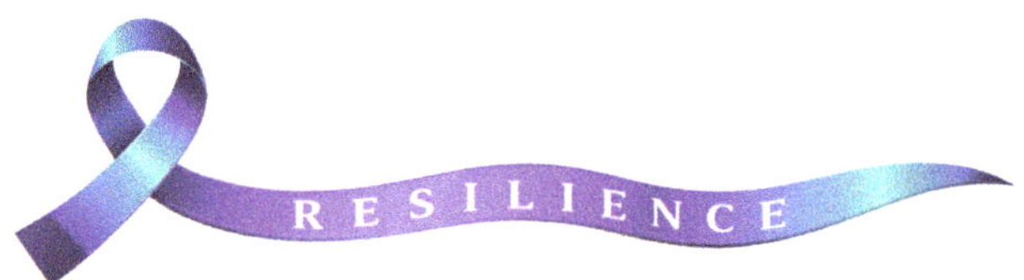

THOUGHTS AND NOTES

THOUGHTS AND NOTES

Chapter 1

GOOGLE WITH PURPOSE, NOT PANIC

Dr. Google doesn't know your story.

GOOGLE. OR, FOR MANY OF US WITH CANCER, Dr. Google. I wonder how I survived before 1998 when Google didn't exist? Today, my world revolves around using Google to search for answers. I'm a learner by nature, and as they say, "inquiring minds want to know."

This chapter focuses on how to use Google with purpose and how to avoid going down a rabbit hole of information that could be useless and inaccurate. The average person desires a quick, easy answer from Google. I'm no different. There is a skill to identifying credible articles, and in the next few pages I will share tips on how to search for information that is likely to be most accurate. Bear in mind, there are no peer reviews or monitoring of content on the internet, so let's discuss how to get the most accurate information from Dr. Google.

Before we go there, I want to share the errors I made when I got the news that I had triple-negative breast cancer (TNBC). I drove home like a crazy woman because I couldn't wait to access Google to find out more about this diagnosis. Not being thoughtful in my search, I ended up spending hours reading all kinds of information that truly scared the hell out of me. By nightfall, my confidence in beating the cancer had sunk into darkness, just like the evening sun.

The following day, I realized the more I read, the more confused I became because of the inconsistencies between articles. One site had me believing I had little chance of surviving this cancer, and another touted great progress in treating TNBC. Or had I read the information accurately? After all, it was filled with medical terminology that was far beyond my comprehension. And I couldn't remember if the doctor had told me the stage of my cancer.

I talked with friends about my diagnosis and cried until I ran out of tears as I quoted all the statistics of minimal chances for a full recovery and short life expectancy. I was convinced I wouldn't be around long because the statistics seemed to be against me. What I failed to realize at the time was that I didn't have enough accurate information to even begin to determine which statistics applied to me. Plus, some of the information I read was more than ten years old.

In retrospect, I could have saved myself many tears and sleepless nights had I paid attention to the dates of the articles and the source; an important lesson when using Google. People tend to upload documents and never remove them, so some information is outdated and no longer relevant. You can imagine how many medical advancements can happen in just a few years.

My advice is to use Google as a resource and your doctor as the truth center about your illness. We humans are all different, and Google is incapable of knowing all the intricacies of our individual diagnoses. Any one of us can post anything out there, and it could be wrong or misleading. You should never consider the information you're reading as the gospel. The best use of Google is to help identify the questions you should be asking when you meet with your medical team, then let them give you the answers and options.

Here are some tips on how to use Google, or any other search engine, to your advantage when learning more about your diagnosis and treatments.

START WITH TRUSTED SOURCES.

Key to searching for information, and the reason I talk about this first, is the need to use only reputable sites. Include the word "research" in your search terms so you're not exposed to blogs or experience-related articles. The following is not an all-inclusive list, but examples of reputable websites:

- Your medical provider's medical institution
- American Cancer Society
- MD Anderson Cancer Center
- Mayo Clinic
- Cleveland Clinic
- City of Hope Cancer Center

DON'T GO DOWN THE RABBIT HOLE.

Set a time limit for searching. There's so much information out there that it's easy to become overwhelmed, which in turn increases your anxiety. It's also difficult to avoid letting your search spiral into worst-case scenarios, which might not apply to you at all.

SYMPTOMS ARE VAGUE FOR A REASON.

What you are reading is a generic version of your illness. Google doesn't know your full story. The same symptom can mean many different things, from minor to serious. Only your medical team can properly narrow it down.

AVOID DR. GOOGLE DIAGNOSIS TEMPTATION.

Use your search time on Dr. Google to identify better questions to ask at your appointments, not to self-diagnose or override decisions by your medical team. I've come to learn that the most important skill when battling cancer is to have meaningful questions to help you prepare for changes and the future. Trying to self-diagnose and determine your best treatment is the worst use of your time.

FORUMS ARE A MIXED BAG.

Blogs, patient forums, YouTube stories, or any other open platform where people share their stories can offer emotional support, but they're anecdotal and highly individualized. What happened to someone else may not reflect what's in store for you. I address this a little later in the book about how to tease out information that might provide value and let the rest of the content disappear into the ethereal world.

CHECK THE PUBLICATION DATE.

Medical breakthroughs and research information change daily. Check the publication dates on the articles or studies you are reading. Stick with information that is no more than two years old. Technology and medical research evolve quickly, and reading old information can cause undue concern and trauma.

1. Enter your search terms.
2. Locate the **Tools** ▼ option below the search field.
3. Click on the drop-down sub-menu and click the ▶ right of **Any time**.
4. Select the date range for your search.

SHARE YOUR FINDINGS WITH YOUR MEDICAL TEAM.

If you find information that concerns you or creates more questions, take it to your medical team. A good medical provider will welcome your curiosity and help clarify facts. Bottom line: Don't let Google or other search engines steal your peace of mind.

PATIENT PORTALS.

While I'm sharing information about online resources, I'd like to spend a few minutes on the patient portals that many medical institutions offer. The beauty of patient portals is that we have access to our medical information, including the schedule of appointments (and there will be many), test results, allergies, medications, immunization dates, and appointment summaries.

Test result postings can be good and bad. Test results are in medical lingo. I have spent too many hours looking up medical terminology while trying to understand test results, and this time was never effective. I knew less than before I started. Sure, take a few minutes to skim the results, but wait until you speak with your medical team member before you let anxiety take over. Let your medical team interpret the results for you.

There is no way to avoid anxiety when you've been told you have cancer, especially when you're still unclear about the details of your diagnosis. Be kind to yourself and know where to look for valid, research-based information, and, most of all, when to take a break and let your medical team do the hard work. After all, this is their area of expertise.

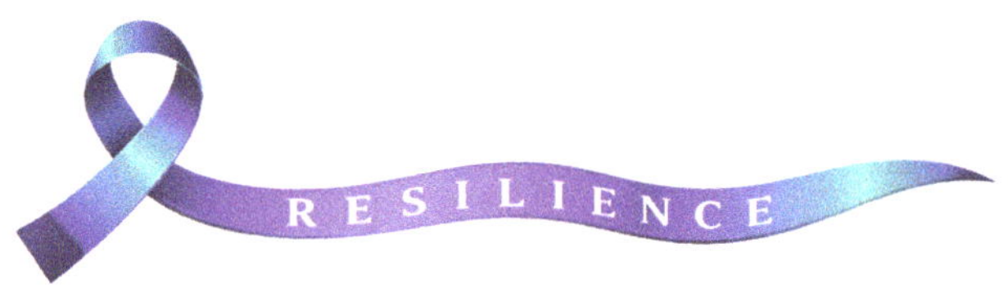

If you are depressed, you are living in the past.
If you are anxious, you are living in the future.
If you are at peace, you are living in the present.

– Attributed to Lao Tzu

Reflection Questions

One way to get started is to consider your personality style and behaviors you need to keep on your radar screen before using Google or any other search engine. Take a few minutes to respond to the following questions and note ways you will try to avoid the pitfalls of unreflective use of Google.

1. What brings you peace of mind during turbulent times?

2. What are ways you can minimize searching for worst-case scenarios? (e.g., avoid using negative or scary words or reading outdated material)

3. What heightens your anxiety now that you've been diagnosed?

4. What ideas do you have of ways to minimize your level of anxiety?

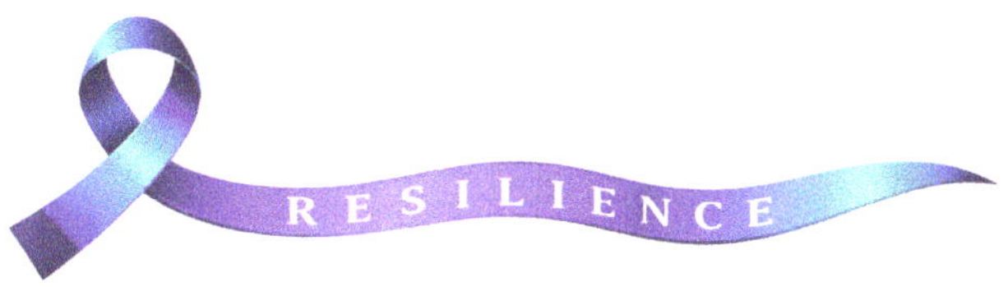

In the first few weeks after each diagnosis, I immersed myself in research. I needed to understand the terrain I had just been dropped into. I Googled, read, asked questions, and gathered everything I could about what might lie ahead. I was in control of the information—deciding what to pursue, how much to take in, and when to pause.

Then the journey shifted dramatically. Almost overnight, the flow reversed. Information began rushing toward me with urgency and emotion—from doctors, from loved ones, from well-meaning voices near and far. Managing the flood of incoming advice, opinions, and stories became an entirely different challenge. It was no longer about seeking information; it was about filtering it, absorbing what was helpful, and protecting myself from what was overwhelming.

THOUGHTS AND NOTES

Chapter 2

RESIST THE ADVICE AVALANCHE

Their story isn't your story, but they mean well.

IT TOOK ME A WHILE to process through the denial and anger stages of my cancer diagnosis. Then it was time to start telling close friends and family members. In retrospect, this was like running a marathon, where I left the starting line well in advance of everyone else. While I was finding my pace and peace with having cancer, this news caught others off guard, as if they were still putting on their shoes to run the race with me.

When is the right time to share a diagnosis? The answer: It depends. Consider the different groups of people that eventually need to be informed. For example, close family, inner circle of friends, the broader circle of family and friends, your boss, and work teammates. Prioritize who should be told first, and so on. Consider the message you want to share. It's important to understand that you do not owe the world immediate access to your news. Telling others is not about managing *their* comfort; it's about protecting *your* stability. Could you use social media to reach a broader base of family and friends? You might use CaringBridge, an online platform where others can follow your health journey, or send a group email with blind carbon copy (bcc) so that many people all receive the same message at the same time.

In retrospect, I wish I had been far more thoughtful about a communication plan. I put myself on the precipice of an avalanche, and once I stepped onto the edge, I realized how unprepared I was with my message. I think I shared too soon with some groups of people. I should have known the stage of cancer I was in, or the design of the treatment plan before telling some. All I could do was respond, "I don't know," when the questions came at me. Not knowing made me feel even more overwhelmed. This is also the time to identify who will be your key/primary/trusted person so that you can have more intimate conversations. Who allows you to be your authentic self without judging or trying to fix the situation? Who do you use for your sounding board when you need advice? Who do you choose to be your trusted partner to listen and hold you through this daunting journey? What do you want that person to know right now?

Here are some tips to consider as you prepare to share your diagnosis. Before telling someone, consider what you want them to know and what they will do with that information. Also, think about what they could do if they offer support. It may be too early to give them ideas; however, in the immediate future, you may need help with rides to doctor appointments, meal preparation, transporting children to school, and emotional support. You can say, "I don't know all the details yet. When I know more, I'll let you know."

I started with my inner, safe circle of family and friends. These were individuals whom I knew would be very involved in my journey. It's up to you to determine how much or little to share. Take baby steps. It's perfectly fine to establish boundaries early on, and if necessary, let others know that you're not ready to talk about the details yet. Consider your emotional readiness, and their need to know. For me, this evolved quickly. I had a hard time telling people without crying. The more times I repeated my news, the more comfortable I became in delivering the message.

Think of it in the G.R.A.C.E. framework:

G. **GATHER YOUR FACTS BEFORE GOING PUBLIC.**

R. **RESIST PRESSURE TO DISCLOSE BEFORE YOU ARE READY.**

A. **ANTICIPATE REACTIONS.**

C. **COMMUNICATE INTENTIONALLY.**

E. **EVALUATE AND ADJUST YOUR MESSAGE.**

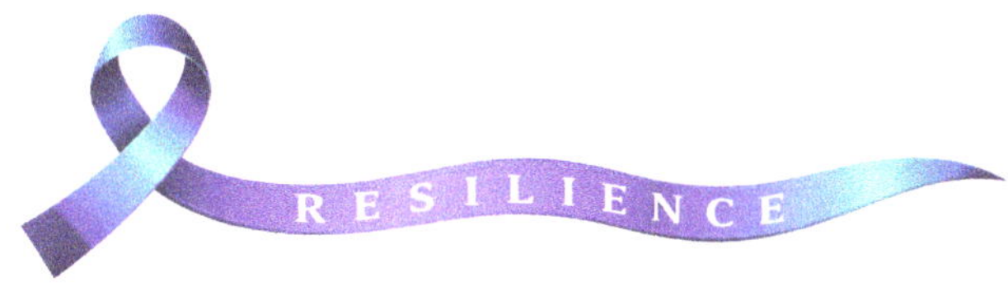

When we're facing fear and feelings of helplessness, a common coping mechanism is to turn those feelings into action, oftentimes through telling stories or giving advice. When I hear sad news, my brain automatically starts going through the archives of my memories to find a similar situation so I can connect the dots between what I'm hearing and my own experiences. That's how we adults think. Sharing survivor stories or advice is a way to offer hope; small ways of offsetting despair with possibility.

I wasn't prepared for what felt like an avalanche of information that came my way. An avalanche seems like the appropriate metaphor when talking about unsolicited advice. While the advice was well-meaning, it was like tiny snowflakes in the air. Soon, the little snowflakes began to accumulate, and as more people added their thoughts and stories, I felt a weight on my psyche.

The desire of others to connect with me and share their own experiences or stories about breast cancer caught me off guard. Conversations often turned into lengthy discussions about progress in treatments or knowing someone who had experienced the same types of cancer and was still thriving. The accumulation of all the stories hit me like an avalanche. It was unpredicted and happened quickly, leaving me without the space to breathe or process everything that was coming at me. Even when I knew every piece of advice being offered was wrapped in love, the sheer volume started to feel heavy, and I began to feel buried under others' expectations, unable to clearly hear my own voice beneath all the information.

It was difficult to hear the common response, "It will be okay. Lots of women have beat breast cancer," or "I know someone who had a stem cell transplant years ago, and they had no problems at all." Like the feeling of snow, these experiences began to feel cold and impersonal, not because the person sharing didn't care, but because their eagerness often overshadowed what I needed at the time. Just like an avalanche, these conversations usually didn't give me a chance to process or react. While the intent was to be compassionate and uplifting, and to let me know I wasn't alone, I felt bad about how it was starting to create discord in my head.

Until I was diagnosed, I had never paid attention to my own behaviors in sharing stories and advice. Now I wish I could go back in time and just listen, give them a hug, and tell them I would be there for them. Yes, I was clueless about what they were going through, and my story really wasn't going to help them. In fact, it may have been harmful emotionally and psychologically. My intentions were well-meaning. I had an involuntary reaction from feeling helpless to *do something*, and that something was me talking.

In the beginning, I listened with gratitude. But soon, I began to have feelings of invalidation because not every story or piece of advice was helpful. I began to feel buried in advice, and it took a lot of energy to sort out what was helpful from what wasn't. It was a significant ah-ha moment when I realized this was my journey, not someone else's. Cancer is like a fingerprint; no two people's experiences will be alike. I needed to figure out how to manage the advice avalanche because I was already feeling like I was short on energy, and it added another level of anxiety.

I didn't ask for the avalanche; it just happened. Going through cancer was hard, and it made me vulnerable. What I needed was a firm footing to try to keep my emotional balance. Advice left me doubting my situation and disoriented about which direction to take.

Comparison steals peace in a fight
that's already hard enough. Your
path is yours, and that's enough.

My first step was to have an in-depth discussion with my palliative doctor about triple-negative breast cancer (TNBC). I needed to know everything I could about what had abruptly disrupted my life. What I didn't know—and I'm not sure too many people realize—is that there are multiple types and stages of breast cancer. I found myself constantly comparing my situation to the stories being told. I soon felt frustrated, like a dog chasing its tail!

The book *Let Them* by Mel Robbins helped me put some perspective on my dilemma. She defined comparison as being either torturous or helpful. Based on Mel's research, torture is the type of comparison that causes you to self-obsess or beat yourself up over something that you will never be able to change. As Mel put it, "Comparing yourself to someone else's luck in life is a waste of your time." But let's be real. We all compare ourselves to others and their situations. It happens unconsciously. The important thing is to be aware that this is what we naturally do and decide what to do with that comparison. Do I let it torture me? Or do I use it to my advantage?

This became my focal point when conversations began. Here's a strategy I tried to follow:

- Express gratitude for their words of encouragement *(and really mean it!)*
- Ask questions to determine similarities or differences to my cancers

- Embrace their information and connect the dots where there are commonalities, or
- Redirect the conversation because we were talking about two very different situations

When someone would start providing advice about, for example, chemotherapies that worked for a friend or family member, I would quickly ask, "What type of breast cancer did she/he have?" (Yes, men are also diagnosed with breast cancer!) This gave me an opportunity to decide whether to redirect the conversation or continue to listen.

Another pivotal moment was the realization that I needed to confirm my own priorities, beliefs, and values. Did I believe in modern medicine or spiritual power? Was I willing to consider holistic medicine that treats the whole person—body, mind, and spirit—rather than focusing on a single disease or symptom? Was I open to trying something different (e.g., medical trials, alternative therapies, doing nothing at all)?

Once I found resolve with these questions, it made it easier to manage the advice avalanche. My entire life, I've been a leader of change, and in many instances, I've struggled with the "shiny penny" versus the tried-and-true. For example, a dear friend who invested hours in researching health-related issues suggested I investigate hyperbaric oxygen therapy (HBOT), which has proven to enhance immune functions. When moments like this happened, I discussed options with my medical team and asked what they knew about the topic. Would they be willing to research and get back to me? Fortunately, my medical team was part of a highly recognized research hospital, so they treated me like no idea was a stupid idea.

The same happened when I was diagnosed with MDS, and the only option was to have an allogeneic stem cell transplant. When telling people I was having a stem cell transplant (also referred to as a bone marrow transplant), so many people knew of someone who had gone through a transplant. However, when I asked whether they were transplanted with stem cells from a donor or had their own stem cells infused back into their body, it was most often with their own stem cells, which is called autologous. (It never hurts to know a few big words, right?)

As you can imagine, receiving your own stem cells has fewer risks than receiving cells from a donor. In my case, my cells were donated by a non-US resident. (I'm still waiting for my Scottish accent to develop since my ancestry was mostly from Scotland!) The key risk with an allogeneic transplant (yes, another big word) is the likelihood of the new, foreign cells attacking the recipient's body.

As I did with breast cancer, I would immediately ask if they knew where the stem cells came from, and if they were their own, I would quickly inform them we were talking about two very different kinds of transplants.

Everyone has a story they think helps you. Sometimes it helps them more.

Self-Reflection

Let me hit the pause button for a moment. I encourage you to spend a few minutes thinking about the following and make notes for yourself.

Based on what you know and how you feel, what medical options are negotiable and non-negotiable? (e.g., receiving blood transfusions, using a new medicine, taking part in a research study)?

What information are you willing to share with others to help manage conversations?

What will be your biggest challenge in sharing these with others? (e.g., religious or cultural differences, your privacy boundaries)

What can you do to prepare to address the challenge(s)? What will you say? (Write your script to help you find the right words and key messages.)

How can you approach your medical team to assess whether they are open to new ideas that could be perceived as a challenge to their professional capabilities?

"Daring to set boundaries is about having the courage to love ourselves, even when we risk disappointing others."

– Brené Brown

Give yourself GRACE. What I'm proposing isn't easy. I struggled with this many times because I knew people were coming from a good place in their hearts. They wanted to help me. I felt guilty for redirecting conversations in a way that could have been interpreted as shutting them down. However, I also needed to start filtering information to spend what energy I had on relevant information.

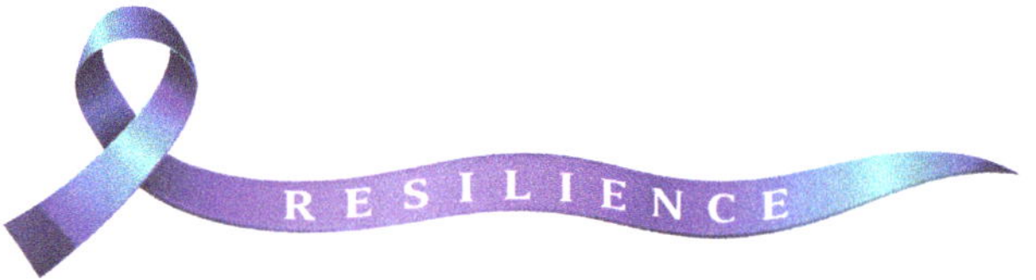

When every choice feels urgent, pause.
Even in chaos, your gut knows the way.

Lastly, let's talk about the advice you get from your medical team. Triple-negative breast cancer accounts for approximately 10-15 percent of all breast cancers. Hence, the use of "rare." During the second visit to my oncologist, I asked her how many patients she had treated with TNBC, and her response was about

10 percent. I had thoroughly questioned Dr. Google about treatments and learned that TNBC treatments are not as developed as other types of breast cancer treatments. I made the decision and was prepared to ask my oncologist for a second opinion.

Lucky for me, she was very intuitive, and after I asked three to four questions about the treatment she was recommending, she asked me if I'd like to get a second opinion. Whew! How wonderful of her to ask. I made sure she knew that I only wanted a second opinion given the variety of treatments being recommended online, not because I didn't value her professional opinion or trust her team's treatment plan. She offered to help me get an appointment with the "Goddess of TNBC" at a nearby research university.

One thing all my doctors know about me by now is that I'm not a person who believes in blind faith. I have an internal need to be as informed and as involved as possible regarding anything that affects me, especially my treatment. A few weeks later, I met with the Goddess who had reviewed my file with her research team, and I walked away with a recommendation for a slightly different treatment plan—same chemotherapy drugs, but two additional treatments and one more week of radiation. The decision was mine to make. For the first time, I felt like I had a say in something that had, up until then, completely overtaken my world.

Taking time to consider both options was critical for me. My thought process went from this is an aggressive cancer, so the second opinion was to be a little more aggressive with the treatment, to recalling all the horror stories of how sick chemotherapy and radiation make you. Would I go for what felt like the right thing to do? Or take the easier path and have fewer treatments?

I'm a firm believer in listening to my gut. Research has proven that listening to your intuition can be beneficial for quick, complex, and emotionally charged decisions, leading to faster and more confident outcomes.

I decided to take the route of additional treatments in the hope of leaving no chance that the cancer would survive within me. My oncologist was receptive to the Goddess's recommendations and my decision. We put my treatment plan in motion, and I had all the confidence in the medical teams who helped provide me with information to make my decision.

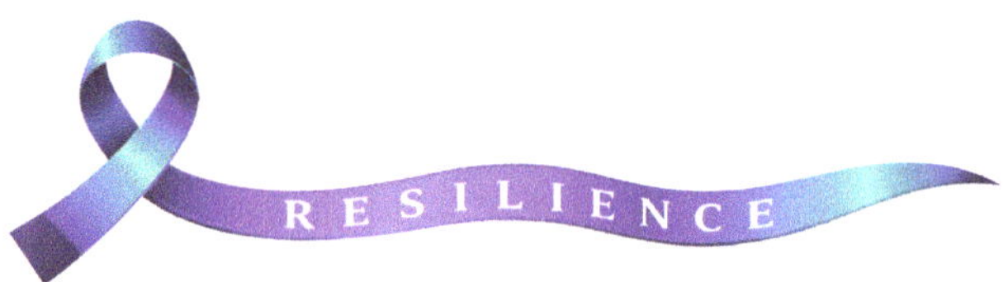

Peter Drucker once said it doesn't matter how fast you climb the ladder if it's leaning against the wrong wall. I compare this thought to the advice avalanche. If I did not manage the advice and stories, I could find my focus on something unrelated. I could potentially waste my energy and time climbing up the wrong wall. Consider the value of ensuring you are focused on the right target and on what matters most; believe strongly in sticking to your beliefs and non-negotiables, because clarity often comes from the ability to manage the unnecessary noise.

Finally, trust your gut, but double-check it with the facts and the advice from your medical team. The way you feel about the path you're going to take can make a real difference in how you get through treatment. It can help you cope better, stay on track with your care, and even support your body as it heals.

Both the avalanche and ladder metaphors demonstrate how easy it is to get off course—by momentum or by misdirection. One overwhelms you, the other wastes your energy. Both remind us to pause, look around, and choose our next step with intention.

ADDITIONAL THOUGHTS AND NOTES

Chapter 3

ACKNOWLEDGE THE EMOTIONAL ROLLER COASTER

Hope pulls you forward, fear pulls you back, and every day, you learn to stand in the middle without breaking.

HAVE YOU EVER RIDDEN A ROLLER COASTER and experienced an excess of emotions? I recall riding a roller coaster only once in my life. In 2019, I took my granddaughter to Knott's Berry Farm in Buena Park, California. She wanted to ride GhostRider, a wooden roller coaster that has earned a legendary reputation for its intense pacing and relentless airtime. Its top speed is 56 miles per hour with a 108-foot drop, and it is 2 minutes and 40 seconds of chaos.

I'm going to try to capture the multiple emotions I felt on that ride because it parallels so well what I went through battling breast and MDS cancer, plus my stem cell transplant.

COURAGEOUS: I had to be brave for the sake of my granddaughter. She had no idea what she was asking me to do. This was all new to me.

UNSETTLED: Watching this ride while we stood in line made me question whether I was up to the challenge. Had I really thought this through? How could I talk my way out of this situation?

POWERLESS: Once we were strapped tightly in our car, I knew there was no turning back, and frankly, I couldn't have released myself if I wanted to. I had to live with my decision to take this ride.

EXCITED: This was a new experience, and the first fifty feet went smoothly. I thought to myself, *I can do this!* This feeling was short-lived.

STRESSED: Once we started up the first steep hill, I was worried about how this might impact my granddaughter. (Who am I kidding? It was all about me at that point.) I was also very worried that I might get motion sickness because I was unfamiliar with the numerous ups and downs and the wildly sharp turns.

UPSET: About one-third of the way into the ride, my stress turned into anger at myself for not finding a good reason to redirect my granddaughter's attention toward a less terrifying ride, like bumper cars. Why hadn't I spent a little more time researching our options before arriving?

HOPEFUL: Toward the end of the ride, when the platform was in sight, I felt some of the previous emotions dissipating because I knew we were close to the end, and we both had survived. There was light at the end of the tunnel!

GRATEFUL: We survived. No incidents. No getting sick. All of the employees did their jobs and ensured that all safety measures were followed. I was especially thankful when the bar was released from across my lap, and I could once again stand, albeit a little wobbly, on the stationary platform.

These emotions pretty much capture those I experienced throughout my four-plus years of battling cancer. The picture taken of us coming down one of the hills on GhostRider shows me crouching down and white-knuckling the bar that held us in, a look of pure fear on my face! I looked (and was) trapped and scared to death. On the other hand, my granddaughter had the biggest smile on her face and had her hands up in the air. She had the ride of her life!

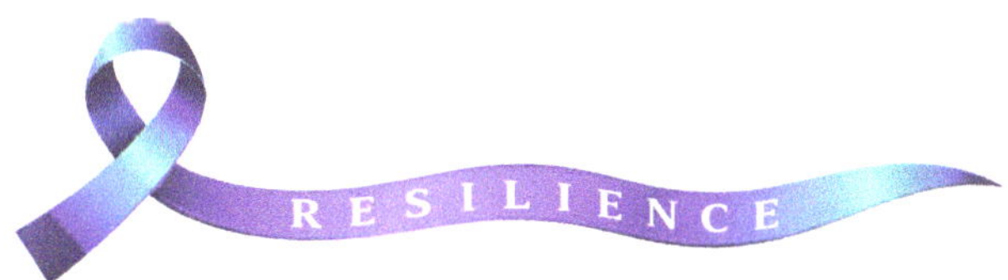

The topic of emotions during my cancer journey could easily turn into a novel. To make sure we're on the same page, let's use Merriam-Webster to define emotions as conscious mental reactions (such as anger or fear) that are subjectively experienced as strong feelings. They are usually directed toward a specific object and typically accompanied by physiological and behavioral changes in the body.

So much of my journey revolved around the emotional drain my diagnosis placed on me, my family, and my circle of support. Every doctor's appointment involved answering questions about my mental and physical well-being. I initially rejected the mental health services offered because of the stigma I attached to them. That was until I finally realized I couldn't shake the doubt and anger building up inside me. I often regret not recognizing this sooner in my journey.

This is where your friends and family play a significant role without your permission. They have a perspective of your well-being that isn't clouded by the medications and other treatments that go along with cancer. I recall my husband coming into my hospital room one afternoon with someone I had never seen before. He introduced himself as a mental health counselor. My husband and the nurses had recognized a change in my attitude and behavior. Honestly, I even noticed I had begun to be cranky and sometimes rude to people, and that's just not my style. Once I understood who this new guy was, I was immediately upset with my husband for requesting this person's assistance. In retrospect, I did feel better after I verbally unloaded about all the things that were making me mad. I'm forever thankful that my husband made the request once he saw me heading into a dark place, even though he knew I'd be unhappy about it.

My personality is to be the strong one and not let others know how much I am struggling inside. One day, my husband told me the names of the many people who had inquired about my health. I asked him what he was telling them, and he responded, "She's doing really well!"

Oh man, was I upset, because I had no idea how he had come to that conclusion. He certainly hadn't asked me! Even if he had asked, I'm not sure I would have given him the unfiltered truth. When I asked him what he based his response on, he said that I looked better and seemed to be getting along much better than before.

It's common for cancer patients to start looking better and often hear "But you don't look sick" or "You look really well!" Because externally you may appear fine, others can downplay the seriousness of your cancer and expect your life to continue as usual. This created a lot of frustration for me because I felt awful inside. Fatigue, the risks involved with getting an infection, brain fog, and the frustration of not being able to do the things I used to do were tearing me apart.

Trauma impacts everyone differently. What may seem minor to onlookers can be something that has a major internal impact on the person experiencing it. This is especially true for people living with chronic blood cancer like mine. Over time, these frustrations became overwhelming. Even when you know loved ones mean well, feeling misunderstood can add to the emotional toll on the patient.

Because I had been on strong pain medications and in a drug-induced coma during the most painful part of my journey, I was unaware that most of my skin had been destroyed (similar to a burn patient) by graft versus host disease.

Doctors, nurses, and friends would look at me and tell me how good I looked. There was a fine balance between wanting to be treated like a cancer patient and being treated like someone who had successfully made it this far. I've learned that the mind can protect itself by not fully accepting and sharing our new or changing reality.

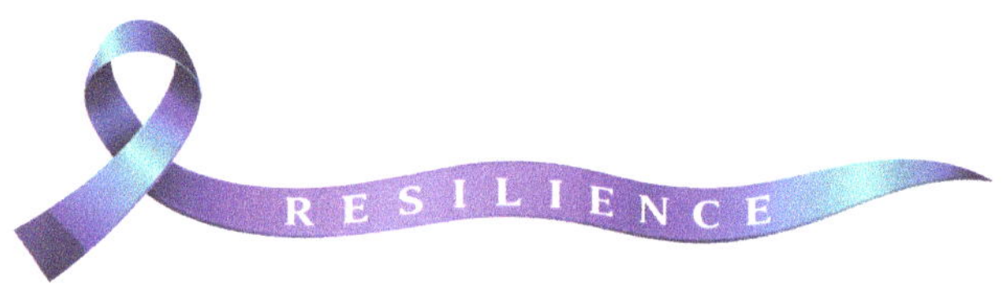

At the risk of sounding overly scientific, I want to share research that helped me understand my emotions and realize they were common. My career had already exposed me to change and grief models, and later, a colleague introduced me to research on resilience and post-traumatic growth. When I explored them more deeply, I saw pieces of each model reflected in my own experience. No single model carried more weight than the others. I didn't move neatly through every stage, and some phases surfaced more strongly and frequently than others. Still, together they offered perspective and language for what I lived through.

The purpose in sharing these models and taking you through some self-reflection is to help you understand that the emotional roller coaster you will more than likely go through —or are going through—is common. You aren't alone, and there are great resources to help you put your personal plan together to battle what is ahead of you—to take the bull by the horns. Insight into each model is included in the last section of the book.

Some of these resources may not resonate with you, and that's okay! What isn't okay is that you don't prepare to help yourself through these challenging times. When reflecting on my journey, I used bits and pieces of each of the models, and I believe this helped me through my four-plus-year roller coaster ride. Remember, we're all unique, so use what makes sense and ignore what doesn't.

It's okay to mourn,

even while fighting to live.

STAGES OF GRIEF

The first model is Dr. Elisabeth Kübler-Ross's five stages of grief: denial, anger, bargaining, depression, and acceptance.[1] These stages aren't linear, and people will experience them differently. You may not experience all five stages, or you may find yourself going through the same stage multiple times. They're general guidelines for coping and should not be thought of as a step-by-step process. Let's look at the stages:

1. DENIAL

Denial helps us to survive a loss. This stage is where nothing makes sense, and we go into a state of shock and nonacceptance, which is a coping mechanism and helps us to survive. It serves as a protective shock absorber.

2. ANGER

This is a necessary stage of the process, so fight your inner-most desire to avoid your anger. At the core of anger is pain, and there are no limits on who or what anger is directed toward.

3. BARGAINING

If only we could turn back the clock to the way it was before. Our minds go through a number of "If only …" or "What if …" scenarios. Our energy is spent on trying to negotiate our way out of the circumstances we're facing.

4. DEPRESSION

Once we realize that bargaining isn't going to work, we move into the present reality, and a fog takes over our emotional state. This isn't a mental illness; it's an appropriate response to a loss.

5. ACCEPTANCE

This is not a state of being all right or okay with what has happened; it's about accepting the reality of the situation and recognizing this is a new or permanent reality. We must learn to live with it.

Self-Reflection

Let me hit the pause button for a moment. I encourage you to spend a few minutes thinking about the following and make notes for yourself.

Think back to a time when you experienced grief. It could be the loss of a loved one or a loss of something significant to you. What was the situation you experienced?

Which of the stages of grief did you experience? In retrospect, what helped you navigate through each stage?

Now consider your diagnosis and where the stages of grief are impacting you. What can you do to help yourself fully address, acknowledge, and move through your cancer journey?

STAGES OF BEHAVIORAL CHANGE

The second model is the six stages of behavioral change, developed by James Prochaska and Carla DiClemente.[2]

1. **PRECONTEMPLATION** (not being ready)

2. **CONTEMPLATION** (thinking about it)

3. **PREPARATION** (getting ready)

4. **ACTION** (taking action)

5. **MAINTENANCE** (sticking with it), and

6. **RELAPSE** (dealing with potential setbacks)

We've all gone through multiple changes in our lives without consciously thinking about how they impacted us emotionally. Consider changes you've made in your life where you were in control of the decision, yet it still created an emotional roller coaster. For example, moving out of your parents' home, starting a new job, moving to a new community, having children, and the list goes on. Every day, we experience change and have more than likely adapted without too much concern. Just hearing that I had cancer immediately set my change mindset into higher gear.

I think it's important to distinguish between change and transition. When you change something, it is almost instantaneous, such as turning a light switch on and off, or being told you have cancer. Your mind is immediately impacted. Transition means committing time and effort to take as much control of the emotional ride as possible to achieve the end result, such as going from a healthy, thriving, independent individual to someone who soon becomes very dependent on others to do basic human functions and to survive.

Self-Reflection

Reflecting on your life, what would you say is the hardest change you have gone through?

What was the immediate impact on you?

Now, think of your process of accepting the change and the transitions that helped you to accept and eventually embrace that change. Consider the timeframe for the change versus the transition.

Now that you've had some time to think about changes and transitions in your life, write down what you think will be the changes—big or small— that you'll experience throughout your treatment. As someone once said, "It's the little things that matter," so don't overlook the entire spectrum of change. What will you need to transition into your new normal successfully?

POST-TRAUMATIC GROWTH (PTG)

The last model I'd like to share is post-traumatic growth (PTG) research. Almost everyone has heard about post-traumatic stress disorder or PTSD, but not very often do we hear about PTG. Post-traumatic growth research shows that some people can and do experience a positive psychological transformation because of a major life crisis or traumatic experience. There are five factors in recovery from adversity and stress based on the work of Lee Gardenswartz and Anita Rowe.[3]

1. SENSE OF SAFETY

Involves not only physical but also psychological safety and requires trust and non-judgmental acceptance.

2. CALMING

Centers on self-governance, a key element in dealing with the limbic system (another big word!) when we face uncertainty. The limbic system is responsible for emotions, memory, motivation, and basic drives like hunger, sex, and the fight-or-flight response; it acts as the brain's emotional center that links conscious thoughts with physiological functions, controlling feelings, behavior, and linking senses to memories, especially those tied to strong emotions.

3. CONNECT

Maintains the relationship bonds that sustain us. The magic ingredient in happiness is connection with others in personal and work life.

4. SELF-EFFICACY

Belief in your own ability to accomplish what you put your mind to and to succeed even under pressure.

5. HOPE

Confidence that even in the face of challenges and obstacles, you can endure and move forward. It fuels happiness and your overall well-being and longevity.

I'd like to think that we all learn lessons after every stressful and traumatic event; however, that's not the case for everyone. This model makes me think of the glass being half full rather than half empty. It's about positivity, attitude, and confidence to overcome the unimaginable. My experience proved that mind over matter was critical to my recovery. I recall changing the password on my phone to one of positivity—*IwillWalk2!*—to constantly remind myself of my end goal. Yes, there were times when I started feeling sorry for myself and could sense the slide back into that "poor me" mindset. Thankfully, friends called me on it and corrected my thinking through reality checks and humor.

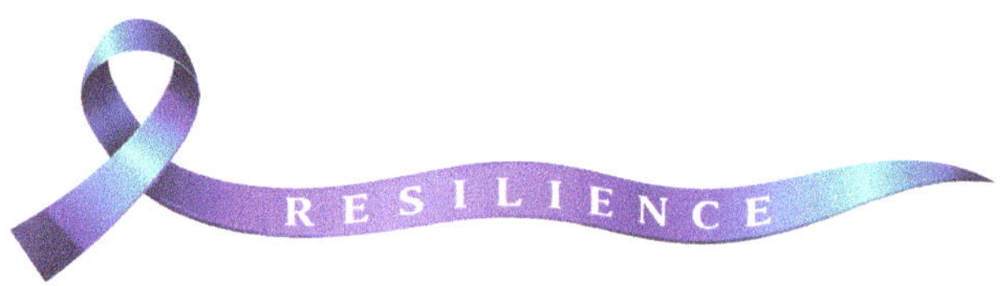

There are numerous resilience models out there, but the perspective offered by Andy Frisella is one that particularly resonates and reinforces the G.R.A.C.E. model.

- Resilience is the quiet determination to keep going when everything feels like it's coming undone. (*Google with Purpose, Not Panic*)
- It's keeping your eye on the prize when surrounded by noise. (*Resist the Advice Avalanche*)
- It's taking the next step, even when the pressure feels overwhelming. (*Acknowledge the Emotional Roller Coaster*)
- It's choosing to move forward when stopping would be so much easier. (*Cling to your Community*)
- Resilience is what enables you to continue when your strength is running on empty. (*Embrace your New Normal*)

What he has found is that resilience is not something we're born with; it's a skill and a mindset that we need to build. There's a link to his website in the endnotes which provides tips on how to help build and exercise resilience.[4]

Self-Reflection

Consider a time when you experienced stress either in your personal life or at work. Consider what actions enabled you to transition through the situation.

What did others do that made you feel safe? What did or could have eroded your feeling of safety?

When you felt stressed, what did you do to calm yourself? (e.g., meditation, journaling, music, walking, working out, gardening)

Who did you go to for moral support and use as a sounding board during times of uncertainty? (e.g., family members, friends, coworkers, customers, social acquaintances, mentors)

What knowledge, courage, and/or feelings helped you achieve your goal?

What gave you hope?

Given the situation you just analyzed, now take into consideration your diagnosis and answer the following questions:

What do I need from my caregiver, medical team, family, and/or friends to create a safety net to help me feel safe? What can erode the feeling of safety?

What can I do to calm myself?

What can I do to calm myself?

Who is in my inner circle that I will go to when I feel most vulnerable and need support?

If I don't have a strong conviction and belief in my ability to beat this disease, what will help me to gain the belief in my ability to succeed? (e.g., resources, ask more questions)

On a scale of 1 = Low and 5 = High, how would I rate my level of hopefulness to conquer this disease?

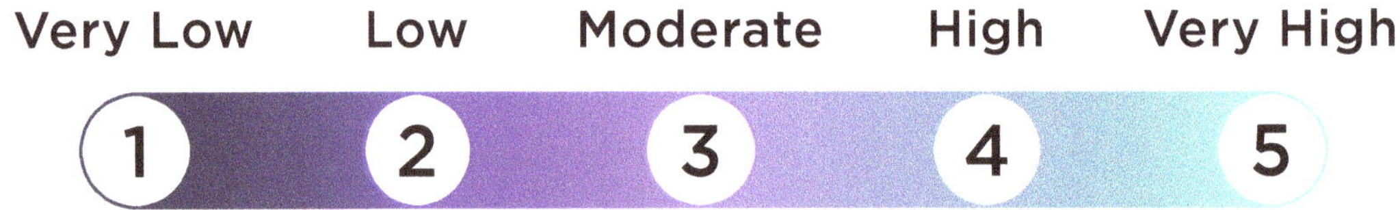

1. **VERY LOW HOPE –** I feel discouraged and see little reason to expect positive outcomes.

2. **LOW HOPE –** I struggle to feel optimistic and often feel uncertain about what lies ahead.

3. **MODERATE HOPE –** I have moments of optimism, though doubts and worries remain.

4. **HIGH HOPE –** I generally feel optimistic and believe positive outcomes are possible.

5. **VERY HIGH HOPE –** I feel strongly hopeful, confident, and encouraged about the future.

If you are dissatisfied with your score, consider talking to your health team's mental health advocate to talk through strategies to adjust your mindset. Most importantly, you must share the above information with your support group so they are aware of what they can do (or not do!) to help minimize your level of stress. Communicating is ever so critical throughout this entire process.

Some final tips and strategies I wish I had known before getting so sick.

- If you're naturally social but feel isolated due to infection risks, talk to your doctor about preventative strategies that could help you safely reconnect with others. Use social media and video conferencing to connect with the outside world.

- Don't be afraid (or too proud) to work with social workers, mental health professionals, or others who can help you integrate your physical and mental health needs into your daily plan. This includes support groups of patients experiencing similar diagnoses who can help validate your feelings.

- Set clear boundaries for those who unwittingly pressure you to act as if nothing has changed since your diagnosis, symptoms, and treatment. Let them know what support looks like for you. Convey your wishes in a direct and kind manner. These suggestions from the HealthTree Foundation for Multiple Myeloma will help immensely in your recovery process.

  » If someone says, "You don't look sick," acknowledge their good intent but clarify the impact on you. Use I statements to express how it feels:

    - "I appreciate that, and I know you mean well, but comments like that can actually make me feel like a 'cancer imposter'—like I'm not really going through this."

    - "Thanks, I know it might seem like I'm okay on the outside, but it doesn't reflect how I feel inside."

- "I know I don't look sick and that's actually one of the hardest parts because I'm really struggling internally."
- "I've learned that appearances can be deceiving, even to myself sometimes."
- "If you're curious, I'd be happy to share what it's really like to live with this."

Gently educate if the moment feels right. Share more if they seem open; if not, protect your energy. Or simply say "Thanks" and move on if that's more comfortable at the time. You don't have to justify how you look to others or yourself. While it poses emotional challenges not to look sick, it can also help you feel better about yourself, even while you don't feel well on the inside. When it comes to lengthy explanations, save your energy for people who truly matter – those who want to understand.

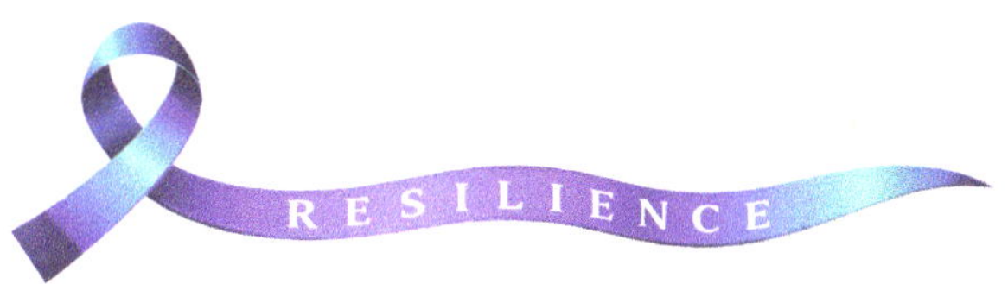

In the title of the book, I reference finding resilience. Before cancer, I felt I was a strong person and could manage any challenge that came my way. Little did I know how much strength and determination it would require to mentally and physically take on the cancers that blocked the path of my journey called life. My experience required me to go to a new level of finding the balance between being strong, yet flexible when needed.

I got so wrapped up in the medical side of fighting cancer that I put my emotional well-being on the back burner with the thought that what will be, will be. My lesson learned was that I should have paid more attention to my mental state sooner rather than later. In retrospect, I wish I had gone through the activities outlined in this chapter to at least help me collect my thoughts, identify where I may struggle, put a game plan together to address those moments, and lean into the areas where I felt confident and comfortable. I figured I could do this on my own because that was how I was raised. I can still hear my mom saying, "If you want it done right, do it yourself." That's not a good philosophy to follow in today's world, especially when fighting cancer. The next chapter focuses on the importance of having a community for support, even when you don't think you need it.

ADDITIONAL THOUGHTS AND NOTES

Chapter 4

CLING TO YOUR COMMUNITY

To need others is not a weakness,
but a source of power.

MY ZODIAC SIGN IS AQUARIUS, which means my personality style is one of polarizing energy and one-of-a-kind temperament. Many resources say the traits of an Aquarius personality are perhaps the most unconventional of the entire zodiac family. We're known for being conversationalists, confident, and loyal friends. One spiritual advisor (Gary E'Andre) says an Aquarius is "community-oriented" and always "working to help others grow," and adds that they "function best when being of service to their friends and the world".[5]

These descriptions hit the nail on the head in describing me. Those of you who know me can stop nodding your heads in agreement. My community has, and always will have, a special, unfaltering place in my life. Building relationships and having a sustaining bond is high on my list of life's priorities. The people in my life—my community—provide me with energy, happiness, and a satisfaction that goes deep into my soul.

I have always wanted to be a helper. An organizer. The person people called when they needed support. I am woman, hear me roar! When I received my original cancer diagnosis—which was heavy, shocking, impossible to ignore—my first instinct wasn't necessarily fear. It was to figure out how I control this. Remember my Google searches? I made lists. I started formulating plans. I reassured everyone else as much as I could. I knew in my mind that *I've got this*, even when I wasn't sure what *this* was yet.

Strength and confidence, I soon learned, don't look or feel the same in a situation where life and death are at stake. At first, I tried to carry the weight of this all by myself. Appointments. Decisions. Managing side effects. Emotions that I couldn't even name yet. I smiled when people asked how I was doing. My standard answer was, "I'm fine," because it was easier than explaining the truth: *I'm scared. I'm exhausted. I'm overwhelmed. I don't know how to do this alone.*

My turning point came quietly and as a result of encouragement from close friends who were fully aware of my personality. I finally had to admit to myself (and to others) that I couldn't do everything on my own. It was time to cast a wide net of trust and need into my community and admit that their support was essential to my journey. For once in my life, I didn't feel like a burden asking for their help. I felt relief.

It took time for me to realize that needing others didn't make me feel weaker. Instead, it gave me a feeling of stability. It gave me comfort. Confidence.

Thanks to the agility and mental muscle of my community, they helped formulate a plan that would continue to evolve over time and play the most important role in this journey.

My chemotherapy treatments were every three weeks, and the week following treatment was always the worst for side effects. I lived hours away from my family and friends, so they had to travel to help take care of me. There were so many new boundaries and rules I needed to learn. In my old way of thinking, they were visitors, many coming to see my new place for the first time. Early in my treatment schedule, one of my visiting friends said, "Jody, you've got to quit being the host. I'm here to take care of you!" Dependence, I discovered, wasn't surrender; it was a new approach. It became a whole new way of thinking.

That moment also made me appreciate the diversity of personalities and characteristics of my community. There are a limited few whom I would feel comfortable taking puke bucket shopping at the pharmacy in preparation for my first chemo treatment. That same individual was at my bedside the day after my first chemo treatment with a full glass of water and fifteen plus pills for me to take—at 7:00 a.m.! She didn't care that I didn't feel like drinking or swallowing all those pills so early in the morning. The instructions from the doctor were to take them at seven in the morning. And she wouldn't leave until she was assured I had swallowed every pill before I fell back asleep.

Not being a person who likes a regimented schedule, I thought to myself, "omg, what have I gotten myself into?" I had no idea she would be this way, even though we had taken several fun trips together. But this was serious, and that was fun. It dawned on me that her empathy level, as described on the

Gallup StrengthsFinder® assessment, was more than likely at the bottom of her strengths. Her approach was definitely more rational and less emotional. It didn't mean that she didn't care for me; it meant she was going to be logical, task-oriented, and in charge of making sure I followed doctor's orders. Ironically, she was with me when the nurse called to tell me that the results from my partial mastectomy showed the cancer had not spread, and they got it all. This time, I saw her emotions come through with tears of joy and celebration.

Once I realized how important it would be for me to consider each community member's skills and personality traits, I learned how to be more specific about my needs instead of making vague requests. I planned and organized for each chemo treatment and caregiver through a new lens. I had to remind myself that I wasn't responsible for everything anymore; it was all about dividing and conquering. It required strategy. Somewhere along the line, I finally got the message from these wonderful women who were supporting me that I needed to stop apologizing for needing their help, because this journey was never meant to be walked alone. We were in it together!

Self-Reflection

It's worth pausing to consider who you want and need beside you on your cancer journey. At first, the idea of intentionally creating a team may feel strange— almost too formal for something so deeply personal. But when you think about who you want by your side through all the unknowns— the good, the bad, and the ugly— it's worth a few minutes of time to consider what types of skills and personality traits are most needed, and who possesses them.

Consider the makeup of any kind of team—football, dance, rowing—where team members are selected based on certain skills and qualities that fulfill a role or responsibility. Let's begin formulating your own team consisting of doctors, friends, and family. Ask yourself: *What skills are critical to have on my team?*

Let's acknowledge that not everyone begins a cancer journey surrounded by a large circle of family or close friends, and that's okay. Community can be created in many ways and through many different places. Hospitals and cancer centers often have patient navigators, social workers, and support groups specifically designed to connect patients with others who will understand the experience. National and local organizations, faith communities, volunteer networks, and online cancer communities also provide practical assistance. And who knows? The people who walk beside you during your cancer journey might be individuals you meet along the way: fellow patients, volunteers, and caregivers who step forward. The key is to remember that support can come from many directions, and it's okay to reach out and accept help from unexpected places.

Here's a list to help you start. Put a check mark next to the skills that are most important to you.

○ Strong clinical expertise and up-to-date knowledge

○ Ability to explain complex information simply

○ Willingness to honestly discuss options and uncertainty

○ Collaborative mindset (not ego-driven)

○ Organization and follow-through

○ Knows how to "work the system" (e.g., insurance)

○ Excellent communicator across teams

○ Helps translate medical language into real life

○ Experience with trauma, grief, or serious illness

○ Practical coping strategies

○ Helps build resilience and emotional language

○ Scheduling and organizing

○ Ability to advocate and ask questions

○ Reliable follow-through

○ Encourages routines and small joys

○ Helps maintain connection to life beyond treatment

○ Supports independence where possible

What other skills can you think of?

- ____________________________________
- ____________________________________
- ____________________________________
- ____________________________________
- ____________________________________
- ____________________________________
- ____________________________________
- ____________________________________
- ____________________________________
- ____________________________________
- ____________________________________
- ____________________________________
- ____________________________________
- ____________________________________

Now consider the personality traits that are most important to you. Beside each trait you select, write the name(s) of those who currently possess, or need to possess, this skill.

◯ Calm under pressure: _______________________

◯ Respectful listener: _______________________

◯ Transparent and realistic without removing hope: _______________________

____

◯ Patient and reassuring: _______________________

◯ Responsive: _______________________

◯ Naturally nurturing but efficient: _______________________

◯ Non-judgmental: _______________________

◯ Grounded and steady: _______________________

◯ Comfortable with silence and difficult emotions: _______________________

____

◯ Calm problem-solver: _______________________

◯ Flexible: _______________________

◯ Not easily overwhelmed: _______________________

◯ Positive but not dismissive: _______________________

○ Gentle humor: ____

○ Sees you as more than a patient: ___________________________

○ Humble: ____

○ Empathetic: ____

○ Avoids comparison or competition of stories: _______________

____

○ Keeps confidentiality: ____________________________________

○ ____

○ ____

○ ____

○ ____

○ ____

○ ____

○ ____

○ ____

○ ____

○ ____

Are you having difficulty identifying someone for each trait or skill you've selected? If so, expand your community boundaries a little more to encompass people you may have initially overlooked.

○ ______________________________

○ ______________________________

○ ______________________________

○ ______________________________

○ ______________________________

○ ______________________________

○ ______________________________

○ ______________________________

○ ______________________________

○ ______________________________

○ ______________________________

○ ______________________________

○ ______________________________

○ ______________________________

Is there anyone who will be a natural part of your community that could expose you to possible risks? Who are they and how will you minimize the risks?

The final step is letting your care team members know how much you value the qualities they possess and share how you hope they can show up in ways that lean into their natural strengths. Regardless of the skills and personality traits, these qualities tend to matter most:

- **EMOTIONAL STEADINESS** – calm energy is contagious
- **RESPECT FOR YOUR AUTONOMY** – they guide, not control
- **ABILITY TO TOLERATE UNCERTAINTY** – no false promises
- **GOOD LISTENING SKILLS** – not just advice-giving
- **RELIABILITY** – showing up consistently
- **HOPE WITH REALISM** – balancing honesty and encouragement

On the flipside, beware of "foul-weather friends" who stick by you, offer support, and are consistently present during difficult times, crises, or personal struggles, but often disappear, become less involved, or act indifferent when your situation improves. It's worth mentioning this when selecting your team because they often become emotional landmines, and the intention is more about them than you. Here are some of the personality traits:

- Constantly giving unsolicited advice
- Making your experience about themselves
- Toxic positivity ("Just stay positive!")
- Drama or emotional volatility
- People who disappear when things get hard

The right team moves with you like steady companions on a long trail, each one contributing their strength, in sync, so you don't have to walk the journey alone.

When my strength ran out,
my community carried me.

A common phrase I heard was "what can I do to help you?" And my typical response was, "Oh nothing. I think I've got things covered." Wrong answer! My community wanted to be there for me, to help me. Some told me later how helpless they felt when there was nothing they could do for me. They wanted to help me through my journey and recovery. I hadn't really thought of it from their perspective. I just didn't want to be a bother.

Take note. You want to surround yourself with a community of people who will speak up and share their perspective, not so much to offer advice but to share their personal experience and provide a different point of view. Once I processed their feedback, I began asking patients, caregivers, and anyone who wanted to share their ideas on acts of generosity. From their input, I compiled the following list. While not comprehensive, it provides a jump-start on ways to respond when others offer emotional, physical, or financial support. Share the following ideas or even make copies of the list in the back of the book and share it with others.

If it removes a task, it's a gift.

THOUGHTFUL GIFTS

- Gift cards that can be used anywhere (e.g., gas, food, delivery services)
- Electric blanket, shawl, lap blanket
- Non-slip socks or lightweight slippers
- Membership or credits for an audiobook (e.g., Audible) plus headphones
- Fragrance-free body care (e.g., hand lotions, soaps, lip balm, body moisturizers)
- Refillable water bottle with a straw or a flip top
- Cooling towel or sleep mask
- Blank journal and a fun pen
- Puzzle books, word searches, Sudoku

QUICK TASKS

- Pick up groceries or filled prescriptions
- Water plants, shovel snow, or mow the lawn
- Walk or feed pets
- Take out trash and recycling bins
- Write thank you notes for you to sign

MAJOR ASSISTANCE

- Drive to medical appointments or treatments
- Accompany during infusions or while waiting at clinics
- Attend and take notes at doctor visits
- Deep clean the kitchen or bathroom
- Prepare fresh meals or freezer-ready dishes
- Organize paperwork, medical bills, or household clutter
- Update social media (e.g., Caring Bridge site) to keep loved ones informed
- Provide childcare or help transport children to events

ONGOING SUPPORT

- Coordinate a meal schedule with friends, family, or neighbors (consider using a site like MealTrain to manage the calendar and avoid duplicate meals)
- Help with laundry and routine cleaning, or coordinate housecleaning and laundry services
- Go for a drive to enjoy fresh air and a change of scenery
- Become an exercise partner to encourage physical activity and provide motivation
- Provide pet care for extended periods
- Keep track of appointments using a shared calendar
- Check in regularly via text without expecting a reply
- If asked, research and share reliable resources for more information

THINGS TO AVOID

- Strongly scented products and foods with a strong aroma

- Diet or "cure" books

- Inspirational clichés and stay positive messages (e.g., everything happens for a reason)

- Tasks disguised as gifts (e.g., let's go for a walk)

- Anything that requires instructions or energy

- Typical questions like "how are you doing?" Here are some alternative openings to a conversation: (see the additional ideas in the back of the book)

  » What kind of day is it for you?

  » I'm glad you're here today

  » You don't owe me an update – I just wanted to say hi.

  » What have you been enjoying lately?

Take a few minutes and consider your own situation. What other things can you suggest to your community to help you and your caregiver(s)?

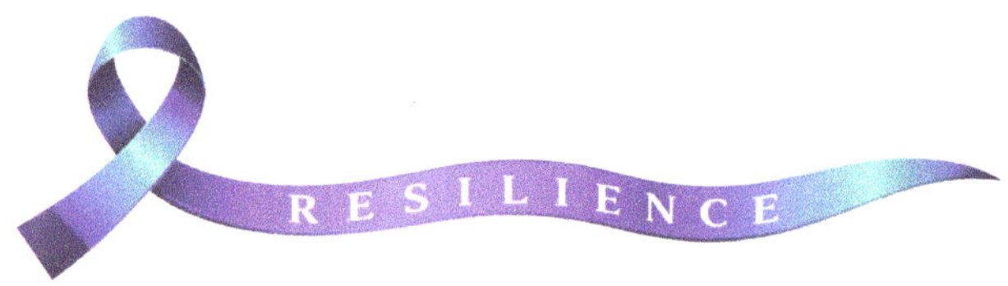

One day, my sister-in-law and I were talking about how often people don't prepare for the unexpected. She's an Emergency Medical Technician (EMT) on a rescue squad and has plenty of sorrowful stories about patients and caregivers who were caught completely off guard when a medical emergency occurred.

To her credit, she put together a list for me, and boy, do I wish I'd had the following checklist early on in my journey. It's safe to say that we're all going to experience a surprise medical situation, and it definitely helps to be prepared. For example, I had a **PICC** (peripherally inserted central catheter) line inserted in my chest, which was used for long-term intravenous treatments like antibiotics, chemotherapy, blood transfusions, and lab draws. One day, I noticed that the skin around the insertion site was starting to look red and irritated. Following a trip to the hospital and the collection of culture samples from the area, they sent me home.

Hours later, at 1:30 a.m., I received a call from a nurse at the hospital telling me an infection had been detected in the culture and that I needed to come back to the hospital at once. That trip ended up being an unexpected six-day hospital stay to address a staph infection. It would have been so much easier had I grabbed an overnight bag to take with me. Instead, I was left to my spouse's imagination and interpretation of the items I needed from home. By the way, a caregiver's imagination and interpretation of what we need could be a chapter in and of itself.

While we can't plan for every situation, being prepared can bring comfort and peace of mind to you and your community. This, again, is where you can tap into your community to help you out. If you haven't already done this, consider asking them to assist you with some of the following items.

Carry a copy of the following documents with you and inform your caregiver and/or community where to find copies if you're incapacitated and cannot tell them. If you feel comfortable with giving them a copy, this will ensure someone has the critical information needed for your care.

DO NOT RESUSCITATE (DNR) FORM. This form is a medical order that tells healthcare providers not to perform CPR (cardiopulmonary resuscitation) if your heart stops or you stop breathing. It's a personal and important choice that reflects your wishes about how much medical intervention you want at the end of life or during a medical emergency.

A DNR form ensures that your healthcare team and loved ones understand and can honor your wishes. It helps avoid confusion during stressful moments when quick decisions must be made.

Emergency Medical Services (EMS) personnel cannot legally honor your wishes without having the DNR. It is not enough to tell them or have the family tell them. For EMS to honor a DNR, they must see a valid, physician-signed form or approved medical jewelry item such as a bracelet or necklace. Each state has different policies, so know the policies for your state.

CARRY A LIST OF CURRENT MEDICATIONS, allergies to medications, pertinent procedures done, and your doctor's name and contact information.

CARRY A LIST OF PEOPLE who can be contacted in case of an emergency. Include their names, their relationships to you, and phone numbers. Be sure to ask their permission before listing them. If you are at high risk of a medical emergency, let them know how important it is to answer their phone—even if the call comes from an unfamiliar number. Here are examples of what to consider:

- Who to be notified in an emergency.
- Who is designated to take care of people/children in your care, pets, plants, and anything else that may need daily attention? Pre-plan for a short and extended hospital stay.
- Who will transport you home after being discharged from the hospital? In addition, include who is able to drive you to and from appointments.

Make sure your address is clearly marked on your house or drive to make it easy for the ambulance and law enforcement to find you, especially if you live in a rural area.

Lastly, pack an overnight/hospital bag and keep it in a place that is easy to see and grab. Or keep it in the vehicle that would most likely be driven to the hospital. Have this ready at all times to ensure you have everything you need when an unexpected overnight or extended stay is necessary.

Self-Evaluation

Consider your household situation. What else should you pre-plan for?

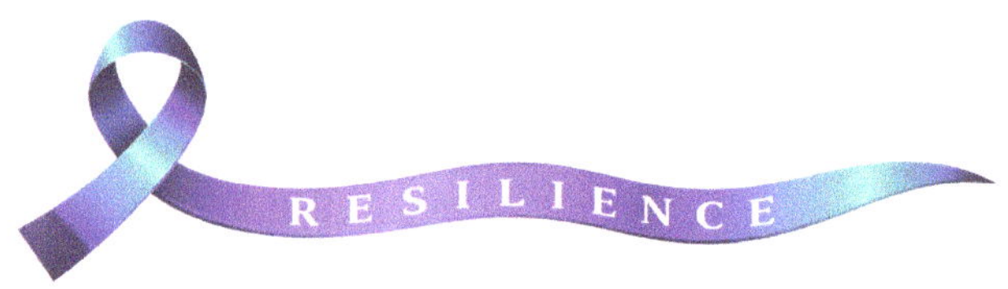

One last suggestion. If you need assistance while at home, find a free volunteer app to help track and organize your volunteer schedule. If an app sounds too complex, consider creating a shared calendar. These can easily be created, and community members typically know how to use a calendar tool.

There are so many moving parts during this journey, and keeping track of who, what, when, and where can be difficult. I required 24/7 care for the first thirty days I was home. This made it difficult for my husband (my primary caregiver) because he had already spent numerous hours with me over the previous five months while I was hospitalized for my stem cell transplant.

We used an online volunteer app called Zelos, and found it was a huge timesaver and helped us keep our sanity … or at least my spouse's and the community's sanity. I still had severe brain fog. Here are some criteria to consider when creating a shared tool to track the who, what, when, and where:

- Community members can create/edit their profiles
- Ability to create shifts that vary by day and time, or allow complete flexibility for shifts

- Allow the community to sign up for shifts on mobile or desktop devices

- Calendar view (by day/week/month)

- Mass or individual emails or push notifications for communicating

- Two-way communication with community members

- Ease of use for everyone. It has to be intuitive!

- Automated reminders and thank-you messages

- Calendar sync with a personal calendar (e.g., Google, Outlook)

When evaluating apps, search for *free volunteer apps* plus one or two key functionalities. Pay special attention to what is free and when costs may be added for features such as the number of users and more desirable functionality. As with most apps, the price increases with the functionality.

We tapped my tech-savvy niece to assist us with managing our online tools and updating my CaringBridge site, and what a tremendous help she was! Many of us know someone like her, so capitalize on their strengths to help you. You'll never regret taking the time to find and set up a volunteer scheduler.

Resilience is built not just from within,
but from the hands that hold you up.

Cling to your Community. This chapter is about finding— and clinging to— your circle of support. Not because you are incapable, but because you are human. Not because you are weak, but because connections are one of the strongest tools you have. You don't have to navigate this journey alone. And you were never meant to.

This is the time to put your superhero cape in the closet and embrace letting others do something, big or small, for you. Let them be a part of your journey so you and your caregiver can focus on you. Allow your community to make your path easier to navigate. One lifelong lesson I learned from my cancer journey is that it wasn't independence that carried me forward; it was interdependence.

ADDITIONAL THOUGHTS AND NOTES

ADDITIONAL THOUGHTS AND NOTES

Chapter 5

EMBRACE YOUR NEW NORMAL

Let the past inform you, not define you.
The future awaits.

THE PACE OF MY JOURNEY FINALLY SLOWED down, and people began calling me a walking miracle. *What now?*

I hadn't worked in nearly three years. I was older, closer to retirement, and unsure of who I was supposed to be next. My confidence wasn't what it used to be. My mind didn't respond as quickly, and it took more effort to articulate my thoughts.

For so long, my life had revolved around multiple doctor appointments and tests each week. That constant monitoring, though exhausting, brought a strange sense of stability. I knew someone was always monitoring my health.

I formed relationships with my medical team and I looked forward to seeing them. When those visits shifted to every two to three months, the open space on my calendar felt less like freedom and more like a void. It was unsettling. I felt untethered … even afraid.

So, this was my new normal and, well, it didn't feel normal to me at all! I returned to a familiar place and faces; however, my life had been silently and drastically reshaped. The changes to my daily routine, going to work, and social behavior were no longer temporary; they were the new standard.

Consider this. We all experienced going through a new normal when COVID-19 impacted how we conducted business, bought groceries, and socialized. Our public health and hygiene habits changed, and we saw the widespread adoption of remote work and flexible hours. It disrupted everyone's world, and we had to figure out how to adapt.

As with everything else when dealing with cancer, our new normals are going to be unique to each of us. Some of these changes will send us into a grieving cycle because what we used to do may not be possible now. For me, it was my level of independence and golfing. The landmarks of my previous life were still recognizable. The people were still there. My values, history, and sense of self all remained. But my cancer journey had me navigating new terrain. Terrain where the ground felt uneven in places where it once felt solid. What used to be molehills were steeper or had turned into mountains to climb. I found paths I didn't even know existed until I was forced to walk them.

My journey led me to an entirely new landscape that was initially very disorienting. There was an emotional and psychological tug-of-war between feeling so grateful to still be alive and yet so uncertain of what was ahead of me at the same time. Strong yet fragile. Confident yet insecure. Highs and lows. Hopeful yet wary. Being a survivor puts me in that in-between space of having an authentic reflection of my journey, yet fighting the fear and reality of a potential setback.

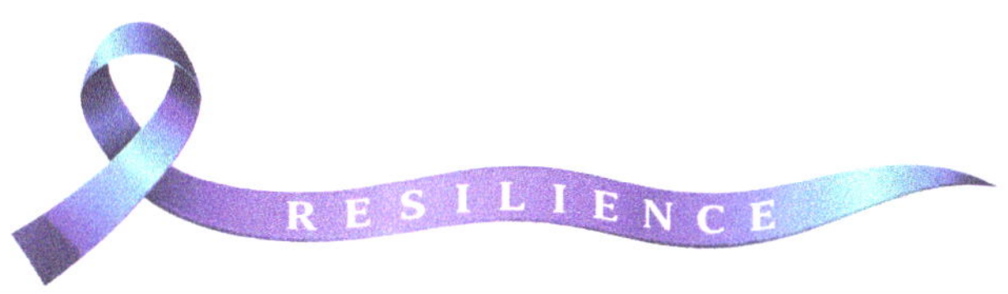

Envision tomorrow, start today.

Navigating new terrain requires something different than endurance or grit alone. These may have gotten us through having a baby, getting married, or moving to a new city. However, thinking I would go back to my previous life—my work, my social life, my family—was as far from reality as possible.

It didn't take long for me to figure out that brain fog and fatigue were now my daily companions. I counted the days, weeks, and months of struggling with these nuisances. I set timelines for when I thought they would have worked their way out of my system. Every day, I focused on denying these two side effects the respect they wanted. Didn't they understand I wanted to go back to work? I needed to keep busy so I wouldn't be worrying about a relapse or a new diagnosis. I missed the social interaction. As hard as I tried, these companions were there in the morning when I opened my eyes and stayed with me until I lay my head down to rest at night. I started to lose my optimism of ever living a "normal" life again.

Then came my stem cell transplant, and my new normal became not being able to walk to the bathroom, feed myself, or sit up in a chair without falling. There were several words (e.g., *#!#%) that came to mind when I realized that my normal was looking pretty grim. How frustrating! I heard my grandfather's voice say, "It's time to put on your big girl panties and do something about it," which I eventually did. It just took quite a bit of time for me to be able to sit up by myself and guide my big feet through those little leg holes.

One of the biggest challenges I faced, besides my physical condition, was the psychological noise in my head—the negative self-talk. I felt a strong sense of anxiety because I was anticipating a future filled with doom and gloom. I was also anticipating another shoe to drop. I learned later that this is quite common for cancer survivors. I mean, how was I to avoid looking over my shoulder all the time when the second shoe (MDS cancer) dropped within eighteen months of being diagnosed with breast cancer?

It came down to me having a serious conversation with myself. I said, "Self, you have to focus on looking through your new windshield and quit spending time looking in the rearview mirror." I needed to put my car in drive, step on the gas, and keep my foot off the brake. In addition, I needed to take good care of myself to ensure I had a full tank of gas to get me through this journey. Afterall, I had places to go, people to see, and things to do.

When life changes the terrain,
you don't need a new destination,
you need a better way to navigate.

It was during my most difficult days that G.R.A.C.E. started to formulate in my head, not as an acronym, but as behaviors. I began assessing my journey, which had started over three years prior, and analyzing the results based on the paths I had chosen. I kept thinking, how could I have reduced some of my anxiety? What landmines did I step right into, knowing full well that I should have avoided? How could I have ever survived without my community of support? What could I share with others to help them reduce their anxiety?

One of my dear friends kept saying, "Jody, you have to give yourself some grace! You've been through so much." Every time we talked on the phone, and I would be crying about my situation, she would remind me how important it was to give myself grace. While grace is commonly used when speaking of God giving blessings and forgiveness to people who do not deserve them, she was telling me to be kind to myself and give myself time, patience, and understanding, just like I would offer to a friend in my situation.

From there on, I set small, achievable hopes for myself. Over time, those aspirations expanded into near-term plans and longer-range ambitions. As my confidence returned, I began envisioning the accomplishments I still wanted to pursue—some within reach and others boldly aspirational. I started with learning how to set myself upright. The next step was scooting from the bed into the wheelchair using a board to slide across. Then stand for a few seconds.

Next, stand for one minute, push myself around in my wheelchair, and so on. I started looking ahead and picturing myself living fully again. I envisioned myself out on a golf course, smacking that little white ball down the lush green fairway. I had to recognize that I was given a clean slate, allowing me to write my own story and select new paths for my journey. I celebrated small wins. I celebrated quietly. I celebrated some loudly with friends and family. The small wins slowly built up to big wins, like walking without the assistance of a walker.

Addressing the uncontrollable changes was so critical to my progress. I forced myself to find the positive in what was happening. For example, underwire bras were my loss because my partial mastectomy incision was between my breast and rib cage. This was a good loss, so I had a celebration when I got rid of all those uncomfortable things. Being unable to walk to navigate my own home was a considerable loss for me. I still tear up when thinking about it. The ray of sunshine I found in this situation was that I had frequent visitors and was seldom alone.

Think about what you have lost or might lose because of your diagnosis and treatment. Have you taken time to grieve (or celebrate) that loss or losses? If not, start planning how you will work your way through these. Use these T-charts to help you identify the benefits and the drawbacks of your new normals, and don't stop until you have at least three to five listed on each side. Keep challenging yourself and dig deep into your fears to identify those changes that will impact you and those around you.

I feel as though I've lost/gained _______________________

____

Benefits	Drawbacks

I feel as though I've lost/gained _______________________________

____

Benefits	Drawbacks

I feel as though I've lost/gained _______________________________

____

Benefits	Drawbacks

Imagine yourself writing in your journal six months from now. What positive changes, progress, or moments of strength would you hope to look back on?

As you think about the weeks and months ahead of you, what feels most important to you right now? What will you do to make this a priority in your daily life?

What are moments of joy and meaning that you want to continue to cultivate?

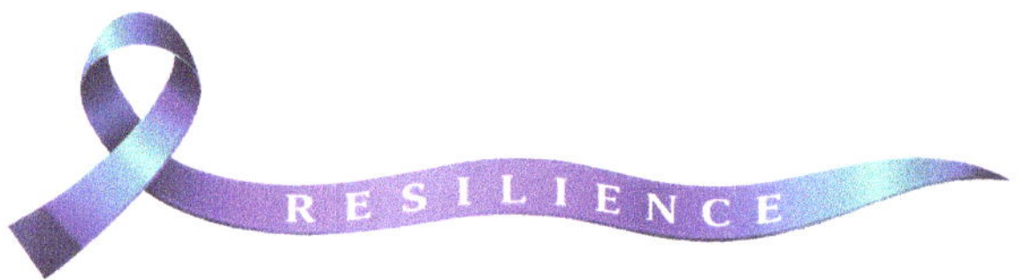

Embrace your new normal. Don't just tolerate it and think of it with disdain. Most of all, do not resist it. EMBRACE it! Whether you like it or not, it's here to stay, and while you may not be able to comprehend why this is happening to you, it does have meaning. Your future is shaped not by what was lost, but by what remains and is ahead of you. Carry forward with intention because there is still purpose, happiness, and growth ahead of you. Envision and embrace a new scenario of strength, where resilience replaces uncertainty, adaptability becomes your compass, and grace guides each step forward.

ADDITIONAL THOUGHTS AND NOTES

ADDITIONAL THOUGHTS AND NOTES

Chapter 6

SUMMARY

Never forget how far you've come. Everything you have gotten through. All the times you have pushed on even when you felt you couldn't. All the mornings you got out of bed no matter how hard it was. All the times you wanted to give up, but you got through another day. Never forget how much strength you have learned and developed along the way.

—Author unknown

WHEN YOU INTENTIONALLY ADOPT the behaviors of G.R.A.C.E., you give yourself tools to navigate every stage of your cancer journey, from diagnosis through treatment and into recovery. Along the way, give yourself space and time for self-reflection. Take note of what you need most to navigate your journey, and practice each tool with intention. Let's review how G.R.A.C.E. can make a difference in your journey.

G. GOOGLE WITH PURPOSE, NOT PANIC

In a new landscape, it's tempting to scan endlessly for reassurance, answers, or proof that the path ahead is safe. But constant searching can make the terrain feel more dangerous than it is. Purposeful information, chosen carefully and intentionally, becomes a compass instead of a source of fear.

R. RESIST THE ADVICE AVALANCHE

Everyone has opinions about how you should move forward. What to do. Which trail to take. How fast you should walk. When you should be "over it." In this landscape, not every trail sign is meant for you. Learning which voices to listen to, and which ones to acknowledge but ignore, is an act of self-preservation.

A. ACKNOWLEDGE THE EMOTIONAL ROLLER COASTER

You can be deeply grateful to be alive and still grieve the life you had before. Both truths exist on the same map. Pretending the emotions aren't there doesn't make the journey easier; it makes it lonelier. Take time to understand your map. It's either now or later, and the sooner you acknowledge that roller coaster of emotions, the sooner you will be able to heal and move forward.

C. CLING TO YOUR COMMUNITY

Some people walk beside you with steadiness and compassion. Others mean well but tire easily or rush ahead. Not everyone in your community is emotionally equipped to be within your community of support. Survivorship teaches you to travel with those who respect your pace, your pauses, your ups and downs, and your need to sometimes sit down and rest. Welcome them with open arms and gratitude.

E. EMBRACE YOUR NEW NORMAL

This does not mean you need to surrender. This is not defeat. Look at it as a change from your previous direction. Embracing the new normal means learning how to navigate the new landscape—when to conserve energy, where to take joy, and how to build a life that fits the body, mind, and heart you live in now.

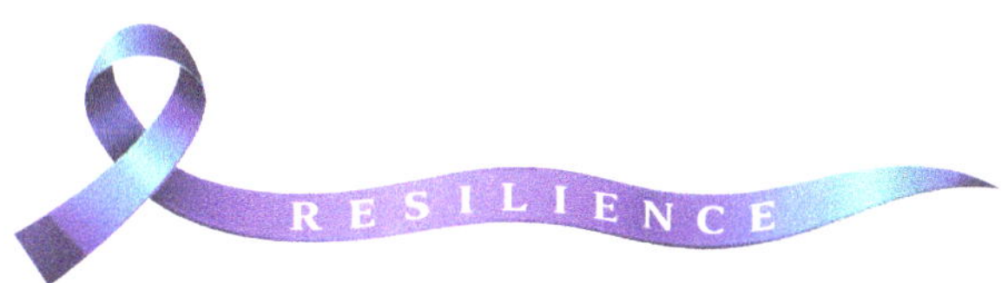

It does not matter how slowly you go so long as you do not stop.

—Confucius

It's time to take a deep breath and start moving forward. You've had the opportunity throughout the book to reflect and evaluate what's important to you. Look back through the pages and remind yourself of how you plan to become more resilient and overcome this speed bump in life. Use your insights to move through your cancer journey with awareness, compassion, and grace— one deliberate step at a time.

THOUGHTS AND NOTES

THOUGHTS AND NOTES

THOUGHTS AND NOTES

COMPARISONS OF STAGES OF GRIEF, STAGES OF CHANGE AND POST-TRAUMATIC GROWTH MODELS

	STAGES OF GRIEF (KÜBLER-ROSS)	STAGES OF CHANGE (TRANSTHEORETICAL MODEL)	POST-TRAUMATIC GROWTH MODEL (PTG)	KEY COMPARISONS
Purpose	Explains emotional responses to loss, trauma, or major life change	Explains how people intentionally modify behavior over time	Explains positive psychological changes that can result from struggling with adversity	Grief = emotional recovery Change = behavioral change PTG = growth after adversity
Focus	Processing emotions of loss and reaching acceptance	Moving from resistance to sustained new behavior	Meaning-making, resilience, and finding new strengths after trauma	PTG looks beyond adaptation, toward transformation
Stages / Dimensions	1. Denial 2. Anger 3. Bargaining 4. Depression 5. Acceptance	1. Precontemplation 2. Contemplation 3. Preparation 4. Action 5. Maintenance 6. Relapse	1. Appreciation of life 2. New possibilities 3. Relating to others 4. Personal strength 5. Spiritual/existential growth	PTG doesn't progress in fixed stages; it's about outcomes and shifts in perspective
Starting Point	Shock, denial, resisting reality	Lack of awareness or readiness	Trauma or crisis as a catalyst	All begin with disruption, but PTG assumes growth potential
Middle Experience	Emotional turmoil (anger, bargaining, depression)	Cognitive-emotional struggle, planning, commitment	Deep reflection, reevaluating priorities, identity shifts	Grief/change focus on coping; PTG focuses on meaning-making
Turning Point	Acceptance of new reality	Action stage (taking concrete steps)	Recognition of new strengths and perspectives	PTG goes further, seeing trauma as a source of growth
End Goal	Peace with new reality	Sustained change and resilience	Transformation, enhanced life meaning, greater resilience	PTG expands beyond survival or adaptation to thriving
Relapse / Regression	Not formally included, but common	Explicitly includes relapse as part of change cycle	Growth is not linear; setbacks can still occur	All models allow for setbacks, but PTG frames them as part of the growth process

FIGURE 2:
STAGES OF GRIEF VS STAGES OF CHANGE: OVERLAPS AND DIFFERENCES

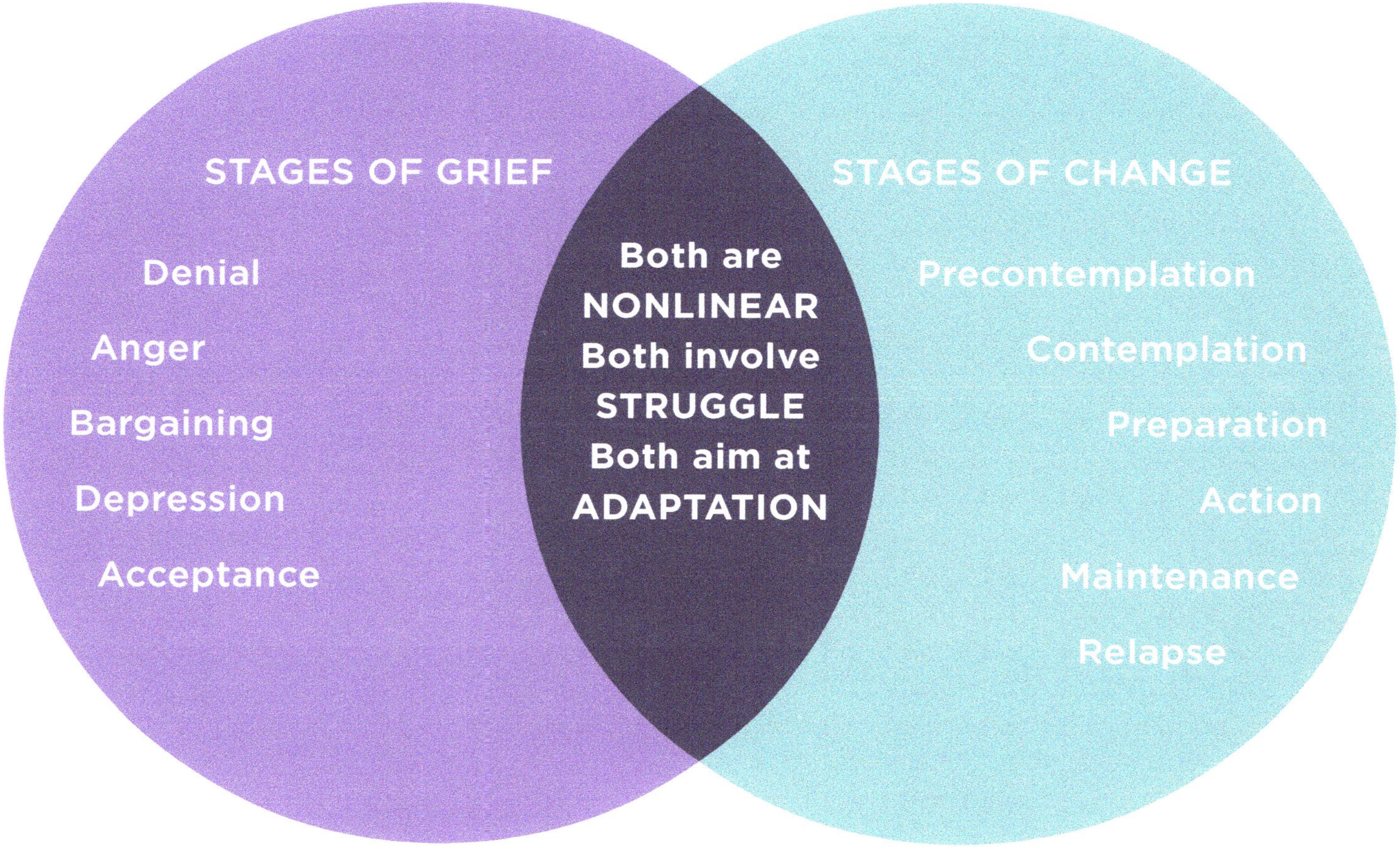

Tips for Community: What to Say/What Not to Say

Your presence is more important than having the perfect words to say. With that said, we're often at a loss for what to say. If you're unsure, lead with kindness and give the cancer patient the choice to share—or not. Support doesn't come from having the right phrases memorized. It comes from showing up, listening more than speaking, and letting the person with cancer set the tone.

INSTEAD OF SAYING …	TRY SAYING …	WHY IT HELPS
"How are you doing?"	**"It's really good to see you."**	Removes pressure to explain or summarize their health.
"How are you feeling?"	**"What kind of day is it for you?"**	Acknowledges variability without demanding detail.
"Are you better yet?"	**"I'm thinking about you."**	Avoids implying there's a timeline or finish line.
"You look great!"	**"I'm glad you're here today."**	Keeps the focus on connection, not appearance.
"How's treatment going?"	**"Would you like to talk about health stuff, or not today?"**	Gives them control over the conversation.
"At least you caught it early."	**"This is a lot to carry."**	Validates experience without minimizing it.
"Everything happens for a reason."	**"I don't have the right words, but I care."**	Avoids platitudes; honors uncertainty.
"You're so strong."	**"You've been showing up the best you can."**	Recognizes effort without forcing a strength narrative.

INSTEAD OF SAYING …	TRY SAYING …	WHY IT HELPS
"Let me know if you need anything."	**"Would it help if I did this?"**	Turns vague offers into real support.
"I know exactly how you feel."	**"I can't fully understand, but I'm here."**	Respects their unique experience.
"Any updates?"	**"No need to update me—just wanted to say hi."**	Removes the feeling of obligation.
"Are you scared?"	**"How can I support you right now?"**	Centers on care, not emotion extraction.

Tips for Community: Thoughtful Ways to Help Someone with Cancer

THOUGHTFUL GIFTS

- Gift cards that can be used anywhere (e.g., gas, food, delivery services)
- Electric blanket, shawl, lap blanket
- Non-slip socks or lightweight slippers
- Cooling towel or sleep mask
- Membership or credits for an audiobook (e.g., Audible) plus headphones
- Fragrance-free body care (e.g., hand lotions, soaps, lip balm, body moisturizers)
- Refillable water bottle with a straw or a flip top
- Blank journal and a fun pen
- Puzzle books, word searches, Sudoku

MAJOR ASSISTANCE

- Drive to medical appointments or treatments
- Accompany during infusions or while waiting at clinics
- Deep clean the kitchen or bathroom
- Prepare fresh meals or freezer-ready dishes
- Attend and take notes at doctor visits
- Organize paperwork, medical bills, or household clutter
- Update social media (e.g., Caring Bridge site) to keep loved ones informed
- Provide childcare or help transport children to events

QUICK TASKS

- Pick up groceries or filled prescriptions
- Water plants, shovel snow, or mow the lawn
- Walk or feed pets
- Take out trash and recycling bins
- Write thank you notes for you to sign

ONGOING SUPPORT

- Coordinate a meal schedule with friends, family, or neighbors (consider using a site like MealTrain to manage the calendar and avoid duplicate meals)
- Help with laundry and routine cleaning, or coordinate housecleaning and laundry services
- Go for a drive to enjoy fresh air and a change of scenery
- Become an exercise partner to encourage physical activity and provide motivation
- Provide pet care for extended periods
- Keep track of appointments using a shared calendar
- Check in regularly via text without expecting a reply
- If asked, research and share reliable resources for more information

THINGS TO *AVOID*

- Strongly scented products and foods with a strong aroma
- Diet or "cure" books
- Inspirational clichés and stay positive messages (e.g., everything happens for a reason)
- Tasks disguised as gifts (e.g., let's go for a walk)
- Anything that requires instructions or energy
- Typical questions like "how are you doing?" Here are some alternative openings to a conversation:
  - » What kind of day is it for you?
  - » I'm glad you're here today
  - » You don't owe me an update – I just wanted to say hi.
  - » What have you been enjoying lately?

ENDNOTES

CHAPTER 3

[1] Kübler-Ross, Elisabeth, 2014. *On Death and Dying: 50th Anniversary Edition*. Scribner.

[2] Verywellmind. "The Six Stages of Change." October 14, 2025. https://www.verywellmind.com/the-stages-of-change-2794868

[3] Cherbosque, Jorge, Lee Gardenswartz, and Anita Rowe. 2022. *Emotional Intelligence and Diversity Series: EID Resilience Tool Kit*. E/I/D/I.

[4] Andy Frisella, "What Does it Mean to Be Resilient?" AndyFriesella.com (blog). October 03, 2025. https://andyfrisella.com/blogs/articles/what-does-it-mean-to-be-resilient

CHAPTER 4

[5] Today.com. "Aquarius Zodiac Sign: Personality Traits, Love Compatibility and More." September 30, 2025. https://www.today.com/life/astrology/aquarius-traits-personality-rcna67276

ABOUT THE AUTHOR

JODY FORD IS A FIGHTER, A SURVIVOR, AND A GUIDE for those navigating one of life's most difficult journeys. While she built a successful career as a global leader in change management and professional development, it was her battle with life-threatening health challenges that defined her greatest work.

Having walked through the emotional chaos of diagnosis, treatment, and recovery, Jody understands the peaks and valleys of fear, resilience, and hope. Drawing on decades of experience helping others navigate the unknown—and her own hard-won personal challenges—she offers practical tools and grounded encouragement for those facing the unimaginable.

A wife, mother, grandmother, and friend, Jody is the steady presence you want in your corner when life gets tough. She holds a strong belief that there is always a way forward, and she's there to inspire you to take your first steps.